Mcqs in
Applied Basic Science
for Basic Surgical Training

S Jacob MB BS MS
Senior Lecturer, Department of Biomedical Science,
University of Sheffield,
Sheffield, UK

R C Samuel BSc (Hons) MB ChB
Senior House Officer
Leeds General Infirmary,
Leeds, UK

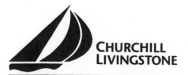

CHURCHILL
LIVINGSTONE

EDINBURGH LONDON NEW YORK PHILADELPHIA ST LOUIS SYDNEY TORONTO
2000

CHURCHILL LIVINGSTONE
An imprint of Elsevier Limited

First published 2000
Reprinted 2004, 2005, 2006

ISBN 0 443 063494

British Library Cataloguing in Publication Data
A catalogue record for this book is available from the British Library

Library of Congress Cataloging in Publication Data
A catalog record for this book is available from the Library of Congress

Notice
Medical knowledge is constantly changing. Standard safety precautions must be
followed, but as new research and clinical experience broaden our knowledge, changes
in treatment and drug therapy may become necessary or appropriate. Readers are
advised to check the most current product information provided by the manufacturer
of each drug to be administered to verify the recommended dose, the method and
duration of administration, and contraindications. It is the responsibility of the
practitioner, relying on experience and knowledge of the patient, to determine dosages
and the best treatment for each individual patient. Neither the Publisher nor the
editors/contributor assumes any liability for any injury and/or damage to persons or
property arising from this publication.

The Publisher

 your source for books,
journals and multimedia
in the health sciences
www.elsevierhealth.com

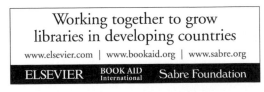

Working together to grow
libraries in developing countries

www.elsevier.com | www.bookaid.org | www.sabre.org

ELSEVIER   BOOK AID International   Sabre Foundation

The
Publisher's
policy is to use
paper manufactured
from sustainable forests

Typeset by IMH (Cartif), Loanhead, Scotland
Printed and bound by Antony Rowe Ltd., Chippenham, Wilts

Preface

The book contains over 300 multiple choice questions in applied basic science, with full explanatory answers, relevant to surgical practice. It is divided into subject chapters which correspond to those in *Applied Basic Science for Basic Surgical Training* (Churchill Livingstone, 2000) edited by Mr Andrew Raftery. The questions and answers are aimed to complement the descriptive account of the topics dealt with in that textbook. There are questions in anatomy, physiology and pathology. All the questions take the form of a stem with five branches which must be answered true or false. The format of these are similar to those asked in the examinations of the Royal Colleges of Surgeons (MRCS) in the United Kingdom. About 30% of the questions in these examinations are on applied basic science.

A book like this can assist in the learning and preparation for examinations. A topic, such as the alimentary system, should be studied in the textbook and the knowledge consolidated by answering questions in this book; the process thus facilitating self-assessment and review. It is hoped that the proper use of this book will enable the reader to build up confidence in his or her knowledge of basic science.

Sheffield 2000   S.J.

Contents

1. Cellular injury

1.1 **Cellular injury is characterized by:**
A Hydropic change.
B Fatty change.
C Eosinophilic change.
D Basophilia.
E Nuclear change.

1.2 **Amyloid accumulation is associated with:**
A Tuberculosis.
B Obstructive jaundice.
C Chronic osteomyelitis.
D Myeloma.
E Alzheimer's disease.

1.1 **A** **True** As a result of damage to membrane-bound ion pumps the control of fluid influx is altered and the cells swell up and become paler.

B **True** It is commonly seen in liver as a result of damage to energy-generating mechanisms and to protein synthesis. As the fat is dissolved during routine histological preparations, the cells appear vacuolated.

C **True** This is characteristic of myocardial cells in the early stages of ischaemia. The RNA content of the cytoplasm is reduced, diminishing the basophilia and accentuating eosin staining of proteins.

D **False** Cytoplasmic basophilia is normal in secreting cells and indicates the presence of RNA.

E **True** A variety of changes occur, such as clumping, pyknosis (condensation of the nucleus), karyorrhexis (fragmentation) and karyolysis. Severe clumping and fragmentation of chromatin together with nuclear shrinkage and break-up is characteristic of apoptosis.

1.2 **A** **True** Amyloid is an extracellular material which accumulates around vessels causing progressive vascular occlusion.

B **False** Obstructive jaundice causes bile pigment accumulation in skin and sclera.

C **True** Amyloid accumulation occurs in chronic inflammatory conditions where there is large production of proteins.

D **True** Myeloma typically has large production of proteins.

E **True** Presence of amyloid plaques is one of the characteristics of Alzheimer's disease.

1.3   Cell damage is caused by:
A   Trauma.
B   Radiation.
C   Poisons.
D   Infectious organisms.
E   Free radicals.

1.4   Acute effects of radiation are:
A   Anaemia.
B   Leukaemia.
C   Erythroderma.
D   Pulmonary fibrosis.
E   Hypertension.

(Answers overleaf)

1.3 **A** **True** This can be mechanical damage or damage due to exposure to extremes of temperature. Freezing cells produces ice crystals and causes damage to macromolecules; heating cells introduces free energy which causes macromolecules to vibrate and break.

B **True** When radiation enters a cell it interacts with water to produce free radicals which cause cell damage.

C **True** Most poisons block intracellular respiratory enzymes resulting in increased acidity, fall of ATP levels and accumulation of free radicals causing membrane damage and loss of ionic control.

D **True** These cause cell and tissue damage by stimulating host responses. Organisms new to man (e.g. HIV) tend to produce violent and life-threatening reactions, whereas organisms which have parasitized man for a long historical period show reduced aggression. Millions of people throughout the world live out their lives in spite of having infections such as malaria, tuberculosis and leprosy. The most damaging effects of tuberculosis and leprosy are seen in patients who make the most brisk immunological response to the disease.

E **True** A free radical is a molecule bearing an unpaired electron and is highly reactive. Reperfusion injury is mainly caused by free radicals.

1.4 **A** **True** Acute effects are related to cell deaths and are most markedly seen in organs such as bone marrow, gut and skin where the cells are normally dividing rapidly. Anaemia is caused by depression of bone marrow activity.

B **False** There is an increased incidence of leukaemia in long-term survivors of radiation injury.

C **True** Damage to small vessels in the skin will cause thinning of their walls and dilatation resulting in reddening of the skin.

D **False** Effects of radiation toxicity will depend on the dose given, duration of the treatment and the volume of lung exposed. Progressive pulmonary fibrosis is a long-term effect.

E **False** Development of hypertension is not an acute effect. Irradiation causes gradual loss of renal parenchyma and nephritis. Damage to renal vessels results in stenosis of the renal artery and hypertension.

1.5   Regarding necrosis and apoptosis:
A   Necrosis is characterized by the presence of an inflammatory reaction.
B   Coagulative necrosis is commonly seen in brain.
C   Calcium flux into the cell is an early step in necrosis and is energy dependent.
D   Glucocorticoids stimulate apoptosis.
E   Epidermal cell death is markedly increased in the elderly.

1.6   The following structures may regenerate after injury:
A   Spinal cord.
B   Liver.
C   Kidney.
D   Bone.
E   Myocardium.

(Answers overleaf)

1.5   **A**   **True**   Necrosis is characterized by the death of large numbers of cells in the presence of an inflammatory reaction. Necrosis is associated with trauma, infection, ischaemia, toxic damage and immunological insult.

     B   **False**   Liquefactive necrosis predominates in the brain; coagulative necrosis is seen in most other tissues including the myocardium.

     C   **False**   Energy dependent calcium influx into the cell happens early in apoptosis. It is passive in necrosis.

     D   **True**   They stimulate production of calmodulin and may influence calcium flux.

     E   **False**   The reduction in epidermal cell number in the elderly is due to a diminution of the ability of the basal cells to divide. The rate of cell death in the elderly is about the same as that in youth, or even lower.

1.6   **A**   **False**   Neurons do not possess regeneration capability. There may be neuroglial proliferation after spinal cord injury.

     B   **True**   Hepatocytes regenerate after diffuse toxic damage of the liver caused by alcohol or hepatitis. However, the architecture of the liver which is vital to its function is not restored.

     C   **True**   Damage to renal tubules can be healed but the architecture of the glomeruli is complex and does not regenerate in the adult following injury.

     D   **True**   Bone has excellent healing capacity and is the basis of fracture healing and remodelling after trauma.

     E   **False**   Myocardial cells do not regenerate and the injured area undergoes fibrosis.

2. Inflammation

2.1 Acute inflammation is caused by:
  A   Microbial infection.
  B   Hypersensitivity reactions.
  C   Physical agents.
  D   Tissue necrosis.
  E   Foreign body reaction.

2.2 Stages of formation of cellular exudate in inflammation are:
  A   Margination.
  B   Contact of neutrophils with the endothelium without adhesion.
  C   Increase in adhesion molecules.
  D   Emigration of neutrophils leaving a permanent gap in the endothelium.
  E   Diapedesis.

(Answers overleaf)

2.1   A   True   The commonest cause of inflammation is microbial infection. Viruses cause death of individual cells by intracellular multiplication. Bacteria release exotoxins which initiate an inflammatory reaction.

B   True   Such reactions occur in parasitic infections and are also caused by tubercle bacilli.

C   True   Trauma, ionizing radiation, heat and cold can cause acute inflammation.

D   True   Tissue necrosis as caused by ischaemic infarction is always accompanied by acute inflammation. The edge of a recent infarct always shows an acute inflammatory response.

E   False   Foreign body reactions to an implanted prosthesis or endogenous materials such as uric acid crystals cause chronic inflammation.

2.2   A   True   In normal circulation, cells are confined to the central (axial) stream in blood and do not flow in the plasmatic zone near the endothelium. At the site of acute inflammation, neutrophils flow in the marginal (plasmatic) zone. This follows loss of intravascular fluid and increase in viscosity accompanied by slowing of flow.

B   False   Margination is followed by adhesion of polymorphs to the endothelium. This is known as 'pavementing'. In normal tissues neutrophils contact the endothelium but do not adhere to it.

C   True   Leukocyte surface adhesion molecules are increased by:
• complement component C5a
• leukotriene B4
• tumour necrosis factor.
Increase of ELAM-1 and ICAM-1 which are endothelial surface adhesion molecules is by:
• interleukin-1
• endotoxins
• tumour necrosis factor.

D   False   Neutrophils, eosinophils and macrophages insert pseudopodia between endothelial cells creating a gap through which they migrate. The gap is sealed after the migration and the endothelial cells are not damaged during the process.

E   True   Diapedesis is a passive process in which red cells escape out of the vessels. It is caused by hydrostatic pressure inside the vessels.

2.3 Neutrophil polymorphs:
A Are the predominant cell population in chronic inflammation.
B Have an average life span of about 20–30 days.
C Have movements that show a directional response to the various chemicals of acute inflammation.
D Are opsonized during acute inflammation.
E Have phagolysosomes in their cytoplasm during acute inflammation.

2.4 Chemical mediators of inflammation released from cells are:
A Histamine.
B Prostaglandins.
C Somatostatin.
D 5-hydroxytryptamine (5-HT).
E Leukotrienes.

(Answers overleaf)

2.3   **A   False**   They are the characteristic cells of the acute inflammatory exudate.

B   False   They live in the connective tissue for 1–3 days and in the circulation for even less time.

C   True   Amoeboid movements are produced by contraction of microtubules and gel–sol changes in cytoplasmic fluidity. These active mechanisms are dependent on calcium ions and are regulated by intracellular concentrations of cyclic nucleotides.

D   False   The microorganisms are opsonized by being coated with C3b and antibody. Polymorphs and other phagocytic cells have upregulated C3 and Ig receptors making the microorganisms adhere to them.

E   True   The polymorphs and other phagocytes ingest the attached microorganisms by sending out pseudopodia around them. The ingested particle lies in a phagocytic vacuole (phagosome). Lysosomes fuse with phagosomes to form phagolysosomes within which intracellular killing of microorganisms occurs.

2.4   **A   True**   It causes vascular dilatation and increased vascular permeability. Histamine is stored in mast cells, basophil and eosinophil leukocytes and in platelets. Histamine release is stimulated by complement C3a and C5a and by lysosomal enzymes from neutrophils.

B   True   These are synthesized from arachidonic acid by many cells. They cause potentiation of inflammatory activity including platelet accumulation. Part of the anti-inflammatory action of NSAIDs is inhibition of prostaglandin synthesis.

C   False   Somatostatin is a gut hormone as well as a neurotransmitter.

D   True   5-HT is present in high concentration in mast cells and platelets. It is a vasoconstrictor.

E   True   These are also synthesized from arachidonic acid and have vasoactive properties. SRS-A (slow-reacting substance of anaphylaxis) involved in type I hypersensitivity reactions is a mixture of leukotrienes.

2.5   Oxygen-dependent killing mechanisms in neutrophils include:
A   Lysosomal products.
B   Lactoferrin.
C   Myeloperoxidase.
D   Hydrogen peroxide.
E   Histamine.

2.6   Regarding features of acute inflammation:
A   In serous inflammation there is mucus hypersecretion from mucous membrane.
B   Fibrinous inflammation exudate contains plenty of fibrinogen.
C   Haemorrhagic inflammation indicates vascular injury or depletion of coagulation factors.
D   *Corynebacterium diphtheriae* causes membranous inflammation of the pharynx and larynx.
E   *Clostridium perfringens* causes pseudomembranous colitis.

2.7   Systemic effects of inflammation are:
A   Pyrexia.
B   Weight loss.
C   Splenomegaly and hepatomegaly.
D   Leukocytosis.
E   Anaemia.

(Answers overleaf)

2.5 **A** **False** Proteolysis by lysosomal enzymes is part of the oxygen-independent mechanisms.

 B **False** Lactoferrin which chelates iron required for bacterial growth is also part of the oxygen-independent killing mechanisms.

 C **True** See D below.

 D **True** Myeloperoxidase acts on hydrogen peroxide to produce hydroxyl radicals (OH^-) and singlet oxygen ($^1O_2$).

 E **False** Histamine is not present in neutrophils.

2.6 **A** **False** Mucus hypersecretion is characteristic of catarrhal inflammation. In serous inflammation there is protein-rich secretion with low cellular content. This occurs in serous cavities as in acute synovitis and peritonitis.

 B **True** This is often seen in acute pericarditis. Fibrinogen polymerizes into a thick fibrin coating between the parietal and visceral layers of pericardium.

 C **True** It occurs in acute pancreatitis owing to proteolytic destruction of vessel walls, and in meningococcal septicaemia because of disseminated intravascular coagulation.

 D **True** The epithelium becomes coated by fibrin, desquamated epithelial cells and inflammatory cells.

 E **False** *Clostridium difficile* causes pseudomembranous colitis. *Clostridium perfringens* causes gas gangrene.

2.7 **A** **True** Polymorphs and macrophages release endogenous pyrogens which alter the thermoregulatory mechanism at hypothalamic level. Release of endogenous pyrogens is stimulated by phagocytosis, endotoxins and immune complexes.

 B **True** A negative nitrogen balance, especially in chronic inflammation such as tuberculosis, results in marked weight loss.

 C **True** There is reactive hyperplasia of the reticuloendothelial system in many inflammatory conditions resulting in lymph node enlargement, splenomegaly and hepatomegaly (e.g. malaria, infectious mononucleosis).

 D **True** Neutrophilia occurs in pyogenic conditions, eosinophilia in allergic conditions, lymphocytosis in chronic infections such as tuberculosis and viral infections, and monocytosis in infectious mononucleosis, typhoid and tuberculosis.

 E **True** This may be due to blood loss (ulcerative colitis), haemolysis (bacterial toxins), as well as 'anaemia of chronic disorders' due to bone marrow depression.

2.8 Regarding chronic inflammation:
A Most cases of acute inflammation develop into a chronic form.
B Lymphocytes, plasma cells and macrophages predominate.
C Granulomatous inflammation is a specific type.
D Transplant rejection involves chronic inflammatory cell infiltration.
E It may be complicated by secondary amyloidosis.

2.9 Chronic inflammation may cause:
A Chronic ulcer.
B Chronic abscess cavity.
C An abscess.
D Thickening of the wall of the hollow viscus.
E Fibrosis.

2.10 Cellular events in chronic inflammation consist of:
A Recruitment of macrophages into the area.
B Production of inflammatory mediators.
C Immune responses by recruitment of lymphocytes.
D Destruction of cells and cell membranes.
E Interferon production.

(Answers overleaf)

2.8   **A**   **False**   Most cases of acute inflammation resolve completely. The suppurative type and recurring cycles of acute inflammation and healing may lead to chronic inflammation.

      B   **True**   Chronic inflammation may be defined as an inflammatory process in which lymphocytes, plasma cells and macrophages predominate, and which is usually accompanied by formation of granulation tissue, resulting in fibrosis.

      C   **True**   Granulomatous inflammation is seen in chronic fibrocaseous tuberculosis of the lung.

      D   **True**   Renal transplant rejection involves chronic inflammatory cell infiltration.

      E   **True**   Long-standing chronic inflammation (e.g. rheumatoid arthritis, tuberculosis and bronchiectasis), by elevating serum amyloid A protein (SAA), may cause amyloid to be deposited in various tissues, resulting in secondary (reactive) amyloidosis.

2.9   **A**   **True**   Chronic peptic ulcer is an example in which there is breach of the mucosa with a base lined by granulation tissue with fibrous tissue extending through the muscle wall.

      B   **True**   This is seen in osteomyelitis and empyema thoracis.

      C   **False**   An abscess is caused by suppuration as a sequela of acute pyogenic infection.

      D   **True**   See E below.

      E   **True**   This is commonly seen in chronic cholecystitis, peptic ulcer (causing pyloric stenosis) and in Crohn's disease causing strictures.

2.10   **A**   **True**   Macrophages are recruited by factors such as migration inhibition factor (MIF) which trap macrophages in the tissue. Macrophage activation factors (MAF) stimulate macrophage phagocytosis and killing of bacteria.

      B   **True**   T lymphocytes produce cytokines, chemotactic factors for neutrophils, and factors which increase vascular permeability.

      C   **True**   Interleukins stimulate lymphocytes to divide and promote the cell-mediated response to antigens. T lymphocytes help B lymphocytes in recognizing antigens.

      D   **True**   Factors such as perforins are involved in this.

      E   **True**   Interferon γ, produced by T cells, has antiviral properties and it activates macrophages. Interferons α and β, produced by macrophages and fibroblasts, also have antiviral properties and they activate natural killer cells (NK cells) and macrophages.

2.11   Macrophages:
A   Are derived from megakaryocytes.
B   Have a shorter life span than neutrophils.
C   Can harbour viable organisms.
D   Participate in the delayed hypersensitivity response.
E   Produce cytokines.

2.12   Regarding multinucleate giant cells:
A   They are formed by the fusion of macrophages.
B   They have more pronounced phagocytic activity than macrophages.
C   Langhans' giant cells are seen in the epidermis.
D   Foreign-body giant cells have nuclei scattered throughout the cytoplasm.
E   Touton giant cells have a central ring of nuclei.

(Answers overleaf)

2.11 **A** **False** Macrophages in inflamed tissues are derived from blood monocytes which, after migration into the tissues, transform to become macrophages. Megakaryocytes give rise to platelets.

B **False** They live longer than neutrophils.

C **True** *Mycobacterium tuberculosis*, *Mycobacterium leprae* and *Histoplasma capsulatum* can survive inside macrophages without being killed by their lysosomal enzymes.

D **True** Survival of organisms in macrophages leads on to a delayed hypersensitivity response resulting in large areas of necrosis by lysosomal enzymes.

E **True** These include interferons α and β, interleukins 1, 6 and 8, and tumour necrosis factor α (TNF-α).

2.12 **A** **True** When two or more macrophages attempt simultaneously to engulf the same particle their cell membranes fuse and the cells unite. Multinucleate giant cells may contain over 100 nuclei.

B **False** They have no phagocytic activity nor any other function.

C **False** Langhans' giant cells are seen in tuberculosis and other granulomatous conditions. Langerhans' cells are the dendritic antigen-presenting cells in the epidermis.

D **True** They are seen in relation to particulate foreign-body material.

E **True** Their cytoplasm is clear because of accumulated lipid. They are seen at sites of adipose tissue breakdown.

3. Thrombosis, embolism and infarction

3.1 A thrombus:
A   Has the same characteristics as a blood clot.
B   Has a laminar arrangement.
C   Has a shiny surface.
D   Is usually not adherent to vessel walls.
E   Shows lines of Zahn.

3.2 Factors predisposing to venous thrombosis are:
A   Decreased muscle activity.
B   Dehydration.
C   Thrombophlebitis.
D   Thrombocytopenia.
E   Polycythaemia.

3.1   **A**   **False**   A thrombus is formed in the living circulation whereas a clot is formed outside the vasculature or postmortem.

B   **True**   It consists of layers of platelets and blood clot alternating.

C   **False**   Postmortem blood clot has a shiny surface whereas a thrombus has a dull appearance.

D   **False**   The first stage of thrombus formation involves the sticking of platelets to the endothelium of the vessel wall. Thrombi are adherent to the vessel wall. In veins a thrombus may have minimal attachment and can dislodge causing pulmonary embolism.

E   **True**   These are ridges on the surface of a thrombus named after the pathologist who first described them. They are not present in postmortem clots.

3.2   **A**   **True**   The muscle pump aids venous return. Decreased muscle activity leads to venous stasis. Prolonged inactivity may follow surgery, trauma or myocardial infarction. The elderly are particularly at risk as they have defective venous valve function in addition to possible venous impairment or relative cardiac failure.

B   **True**   This increases blood viscosity.

C   **False**   Inflammation due to thrombus is thrombophlebitis. Thrombus due to inflammation is known as phlebothrombosis.

D   **False**   Increased number of platelets following surgery or trauma is a predisposing factor. Thrombocytopenia causes a bleeding diathesis.

E   **True**   Polycythaemia increases the coagulability of blood and can predispose to venous thrombosis.

3.3   Regarding venous thromboembolism:
A   The incidence of pulmonary embolism is about 1%.
B   The majority of venous emboli arise in the lower limb.
C   Most venous emboli will produce pulmonary embolism.
D   It can be silent.
E   It may cause sudden death.

3.4   Embolism may be caused by:
A   An aneurysm.
B   Atheromatous plaque.
C   Intravenous cannulae.
D   Fractures.
E   Tumours.

3.5   Small vessel obstruction can be due to:
A   Vasculitis.
B   Microembolism.
C   Cryoglobulins.
D   Thrombocythaemia.
E   Venous obstruction.

(Answers overleaf)

3.3 **A** **False** Approximately 10% of postmortem examinations show evidence of pulmonary embolism. About 30% of hospital inpatients have deep vein thrombosis.

      B **True** They travel up the inferior vena cava into the right side of the heart and into the pulmonary artery.

      C **True** Pulmonary embolism will occur unless there is an abnormal communication between the right and left sides of the heart. Emboli will not arrest earlier in the circulation because the veins increase in diameter with the direction of blood flow.

      D **True** Pulmonary emboli may be small and multiple and can be dissolved by thrombolysis or may be incorporated into the vessel wall causing proliferation of endothelium and smooth muscle cells. Multiple small emboli may cause diffuse narrowing of small vessels resulting in pulmonary hypertension.

      E **True** A massive embolism blocks both pulmonary arteries, leading to circulatory collapse.

3.4 **A** **True** An arterial embolism may arise from an aneurysm, especially that of the popliteal artery.

      B **True** Platelet emboli may arise from the surface of atheromatous plaques.

      C **True** An air embolism is possible but very uncommon and volumes of air less than 100 ml are very unlikely to cause any problems.

      D **True** Globules of fat may enter the circulation following fractures of long bones but clinical consequences are rare. Pulmonary fat embolism is a frequent postmortem finding, although it is unlikely that this was the cause of death. Sometimes the emboli may pass through to the systemic circulation and may become impacted in the capillaries of kidney, brain and skin with serious clinical consequences.

      E **True** Malignant tumours tend to invade blood vessels causing embolism. Tumour emboli are coated with thrombus, rendering them more attractive to phagocytic cells.

3.5 **A** **True** Arterioles, capillaries or venules may be blocked.

      B **True** This occurs in sickle cell disease.

      C **True** This is because they precipitate on exposure to cold.

      D **True** The excess number of platelets block the microcirculation.

      E **True** The rare condition of phlegmasia caerulea dolens, an iliofemoral thrombosis causing severe venous engorgement, may block the distal arterioles causing 'venous gangrene'.

3.6 **Regarding infarction:**
A   Red infarct precedes pale infarct in all tissues.
B   It is surrounded by an area of acute inflammation.
C   It results in liquefactive necrosis of the brain.
D   Pulmonary infarction is more common in the younger age group.
E   Myocardial infarction may cause bacteraemia.

3.7 **Regarding gangrene:**
A   Gangrenous tissue appears black owing to accumulation of melanin.
B   Gas gangrene is caused by *Clostridium perfringens*.
C   Meleney's gangrene is a gangrene of the scrotum of elderly diabetics.
D   Fournier's gangrene and Meleney's gangrene have similar aetiology.
E   In necrotizing fasciitis the overlying skin may appear normal.

(Answers overleaf)

3.6 **A** **False** An infarct soon after formation in many tissues contains blood and is known as red infarct; after 24–36 hours, autolysis removes blood to form a pale infarct. However, cerebral infarcts are usually pale and lung infarct remains red until repair.

B **True** There is a rise in polymorphs and macrophages.

C **True** It may give rise to a cavity.

D **False** Pulmonary infarction is very rare in young people even if a main pulmonary artery is occluded.

E **True** It may give rise to shock and transient ischaemic changes in the bowel resulting in bacterial translocation into the blood.

3.7 **A** **False** The affected tissues appear black because of the deposition of iron sulphide from degraded haemoglobin.

B **True** It is a dangerous form of tissue necrosis caused by the spores of clostridia entering a wound in which there is extensive muscle and soft tissue injury.

C **False** Meleney's gangrene may occur at the site of abdominal surgery or at the site of accidental skin abrasion. Fournier's gangrene is a rapidly progressive gangrene of the scrotum occurring mostly in elderly diabetics.

D **True** Only the sites of infection are different. Both are attributed to a combination of anaerobic and aerobic bacteria causing cellulitis followed by gangrene.

E **True** The initial external appearance of the skin remains normal while the necrotizing process spreads along the fascial planes causing extensive necrosis. At a later stage the skin, deprived of its blood supply, becomes painful, red, and finally necrotic.

4. Growth and differentiation

4.1 Regarding the cell cycle:
  A   DNA synthesis occurs during the M phase.
  B   DNA synthesis is initiated by growth factors.
  C   Fully differentiated cells escape the cycle at the G_1 phase.
  D   All the different phases are variable in duration in different cell populations.
  E   All the drugs used in cancer treatment block the M phase.

4.2 Apoptosis:
  A   Is the process by which a large number of cells die in one area.
  B   Mainly involves lysosomes and lysosomal enzymes.
  C   Is an essential part of morphogenesis.
  D   If termed *histogenic apoptosis*, is a pathological process.
  E   Is regulated by gene products such as *bcl-2* and *bax* protein.

(Answers overleaf)

4.1 **A** **False** Mitosis takes place in the M phase which is followed by the G_1 phase (1st gap phase). After G_1, if the cell is going to divide again, DNA synthesis occurs in the S phase which is followed by the G_2 phase (2nd gap phase) before the next M phase.

B **True** Growth factors such as EGF (epidermal growth factor), PDGF (platelet-derived growth factor), IGF-1 and IGF-2 (insulin-like growth factors) stimulate the nucleus of the cell to activate transcription factors to initiate DNA synthesis.

C **True** These cells enter the G_0 or resting phase, some temporarily, whereas others such as neurons permanently lose their potential to divide.

D **False** It is the G_1 phase which is variable in duration between rapidly dividing and slowly dividing cells. The duration of other phases of the cell cycle remains the same for all cells.

E **False** They may act at different phases of the cycle. Methotrexate acts at the S phase, vincristine at the M phase and corticosteroids at G_1, whereas cyclophosphamide acts at the S phase, M phase and G_1 phase.

4.2 **A** **False** Apoptosis is programmed death of scattered single cells. It is a physiological process by which the tissue maintains the optimum cell number by balancing cell renewal and cell death.

B **False** Lysosomes are not involved in apoptosis. Non-lysosomal endonuclease digests the nucleus to fragments and the cell debris is phagocytosed by adjacent unaffected cells.

C **True** It is involved in the morphogenesis of all organs. Failure may contribute to the development of syndactyly (webbed fingers), cleft lip and spina bifida.

D **False** This is a normal developmental process. Examples are histogenic apoptosis causing regression of Müllerian ducts in the male and Wolffian ducts in the female.

E **True** *bcl-2* inhibits factors inducing apoptosis and *bax* protein enhances such factors. The ratio of *bcl-2* to *bax* constitutes a molecular switch determining the susceptibility of the cell to apoptotic stimuli.

4.3   During healing of a skin wound:
  A   There is platelet aggregation in the blood vessels.
  B   Basal layers of the epidermis proliferate.
  C   Myofibroblasts in the dermis proliferate.
  D   Fibronectin aids migration of epithelial and dermal cells.
  E   There is budding and proliferation of capillaries.

4.4   During the healing of an ulcer:
  A   The healing factors overpower the ulcerating factors.
  B   Angiogenesis contributes to the formation of red granulation tissue.
  C   Myofibroblasts proliferate and migrate to the ulcer crater.
  D   Epithelial cells migrate over the new scar tissue.
  E   Subepithelial myofibroblasts contract.

4.5   Regarding hyperplasia:
  A   Left ventricular myocardium responds to hypertension by hyperplasia and hypertrophy.
  B   Smooth muscle cells in the arterial wall are capable of hypertrophy but not hyperplasia.
  C   Organ transplants produce hyperplasia of T lymphocytes.
  D   Cirrhosis of the liver may cause hyperplasia of the breast tissue in males.
  E   In Paget's disease there is hyperplasia of both osteoclasts and osteoblasts.

(Answers overleaf)

4.3 **A** **True**   Platelets release PDGF (platelet-derived growth factor) and TGF-β (transforming growth factor beta) and these have chemotactic action on macrophages and other inflammatory cells which then migrate into the wound.

      B **True**   The proliferation is promoted by EGF, IGF-1 and IGF-2. PDGF stimulates cells in G_0 to move to G_1 and divide.

      C **True**   The stimulus for this is given by PDGF and TGF-β.

      D **True**

      E **True**   This is promoted by growth factors such as vascular endothelial growth factor (VEGF) secreted by hypoxic cells and macrophages.

4.4 **A** **True**   Ulcerating factors such as hypoxia, gastric juice and infection contribute to the formation of an ulcer. Ulcers which fail to heal after the removal of ulcerating factors may indicate the presence of an underlying neoplasm.

      B **True**   Capillaries proliferate and migrate to the base of the ulcer. Angiogenic growth factors are produced by the macrophages.

      C **True**   They secrete collagen and matrix proteins which fill the ulcer crater.

      D **True**   The epithelium at the edge of the ulcer proliferates and migrates over the granulation tissue filling the whole ulcer crater.

      E **True**   The myofibroblasts are converted to mature fibroblasts.

4.5 **A** **False**   Myocardial cells cannot undergo mitosis and hence the muscle mass increase is entirely by hypertrophy.

      B **False**   They are capable of proliferation as well as hypertrophy. Hypertension produces a hypertrophic response and during the development of atherosclerosis there is hyperplasia in response to platelet-derived growth factors.

      C **True**   This occurs in all cell-mediated immune responses.

      D **True**   This is due to high levels of oestrogen; it also occurs in oestrogen treatment of prostatic cancers. Gynaecomastia can be secondary to treatment with spironolactone, cimetidine and digoxin.

      E **True**   This will produce thickened but weak bones. There is abnormal increase in proliferation and activity of osteoclasts with excessive bone resorption. This leads to proliferation of osteoblasts producing coarse trabecular bone with thickened cortex.

4.6   Atrophy is associated with:
A   Increased functional demand.
B   Nerve injury.
C   Ischaemia.
D   Compression of tissues.
E   Endocrine anomalies.

4.7   Concerning metaplasia:
A   It is a premalignant cellular differentiation.
B   Glandular metaplasia occurs in the trachea and bronchi in tobacco smokers.
C   It is associated with prostatic hyperplasia.
D   It is seen in Barrett's oesophagus.
E   Intestinal metaplasia occurs in chronic gastritis.

4.8   Dysplasia is characterized by:
A   Hypoplasia of cells.
B   Cellular atypia and pleomorphism.
C   High nuclear to cytoplasm ratio.
D   Hyperchromatic nuclei.
E   Altered differentiation.

(Answers overleaf)

4.6   **A**   **False**   Decreased workload causes atrophy as in atrophy of muscles following immobilization after fracture or due to prolonged weightlessness which may occur in astronauts.

   B   **True**   Loss of innervation of muscle causes muscle atrophy; paraplegia causes disuse atrophy of the limbs.

   C   **True**   This is due to tissue hypoxia. Epidermal atrophy may occur in limbs of patients with varicose veins or with atherosclerosis.

   D   **True**   Prolonged compression of tissue by tumour or compression of skin and soft tissues in a patient who is bedridden may lead to atrophy due to tissue ischaemia.

   E   **True**   Decreased adrenocorticotrophic hormone (ACTH) secretion may cause atrophy of the adrenal gland. This may happen in patients who are being treated with high doses of steroids.

4.7   **A**   **False**   Metaplasia is an adaptive response to withstand adverse environmental changes. It can occur in association with dysplasia, which is premalignant.

   B   **False**   The columnar cells of the respiratory epithelium change to squamous cells. This is known as squamous metaplasia.

   C   **True**   Squamous metaplasia is seen around areas of infarction in prostatic hyperplasia.

   D   **True**   Glandular metaplasia where squamous cells change to columnar cells occurs in Barrett's oesophagus. This is not premalignant, but the associated dysplasia increases the risk of developing malignancy.

   E   **True**   Gastric mucus cells, normally producing neutral mucus, change to the intestinal type of acid mucus-producing goblet cells.

4.8   **A**   **False**   Dysplasia shows increased cell growth including increased mitotic figures.

   B   **True**   Dysplasia shows variation in size and shape of the cells and nuclei.

   C   **True**

   D   **True**   This is due to increased DNA content of the nuclei.

   E   **True**   Cells often appear more primitive than normal.

4.9   Congenital disorders of differentiation and morphogenesis can be caused by:

A   Autosomal chromosomal abnormality.
B   Sex chromosomal anomalies.
C   Single gene alterations.
D   Failure of cell and organ migration.
E   Exposure to teratogens.

4.10   Anomalies of organogenesis are:

A   Agenesis.
B   Atresia.
C   Hypoplasia.
D   Metaplasia.
E   Ectopia.

(Answers overleaf)

A **True** Common disorders in this group involve the presence of an additional chromosome (trisomy). Trisomy 21 is Down's syndrome, which occurs in 1 in 1000 births. Trisomy 18 (Edwards' syndrome) affects 1 in 5000 births and is associated with ear, jaw, cardiac, renal and skeletal abnormalities. Trisomy 13 (Patau's syndrome) affects 1 in 6000 births and is characterized by microcephaly, cleft lip and cleft palate, and polydactyly as well as cardiac and visceral defects.

B **True** Disorders affecting the sex chromosomes are common and they induce abnormalities of sexual development and fertility. Klinefelter's syndrome and Turner's syndrome are examples.

C **True** Disorders in this category include congenital hypothyroidism, albinism, phenylketonuria and glycogen storage disorders such as glucose-6-phosphate dehydrogenase (G6PD) deficiency.

D **True** Undescended testis and Hirschsprung's disease caused by failure of craniocaudal migration of neuroblasts in weeks 5–12 are examples.

E **True** Severe effects are produced if the exposure is at 4–5 weeks of gestation (period of early organogenesis). Malformations produced by thalidomide and rubella are examples.

4.10 **A** **True** This is the failure of development of an organ or a structure within it. Renal agenesis can occur because of failure of formation of the ureteric bud which normally initiates the development of the metanephros or 'adult' kidney.

B **True** Tubular structures with epithelial lining may fail to develop a lumen; oesophageal atresia, biliary atresia and urethral atresia are examples.

C **True** This is the failure of development of the normal size of an organ or part of an organ. Development of the acetabulum may be hypoplastic giving a flattened roof causing congenital dislocation of the hip.

D **False** This is an acquired anomaly of growth and differentiation and does not occur during organogenesis.

E **True** Small areas of mature tissue of one organ may be present in another organ. Meckel's diverticulum containing pancreatic or gastric epithelium and endometriosis where endometrial tissue is found on the peritoneum and the ovary are examples.

5. Neoplasia

5.1 Regarding carcinogens:
A Schistosomiasis is associated with transitional cell carcinoma of the bladder.
B *Helicobacter pylori* infection is associated with gastric carcinoma.
C Asbestos is linked with mesothelioma but not carcinoma of the bronchus.
D Oestrogens are associated with hepatocellular carcinoma.
E Ultraviolet light conveys more energy to the tissues than X-rays.

5.2 Regarding viral carcinogenesis:
A Human T lymphotrophic virus 1 (HTLV-1) is an RNA virus.
B Human papillomavirus (HPV) is a DNA virus.
C Human immunodeficiency virus (HIV) does not have a direct carcinogenic effect.
D Epstein–Barr virus is associated with nasopharyngeal carcinoma.
E Epstein–Barr infection and tuberculosis infection are cofactors in the formation of Burkitt's lymphoma.

5.3 Regarding chemical carcinogens:
A β-naphthylamine is associated with carcinoma of the bladder.
B β-naphthylamine is converted into the active carcinogen in the kidneys.
C Smoking is a risk factor for tumours of the kidney.
D Polycyclic aromatic hydrocarbons in tobacco smoke are procarcinogens.
E Polycyclic aromatic hydrocarbons act by alkylating RNA.

5.4 Regarding tumour genetics:
A The retinoblastoma (Rb) gene is an oncogene.
B Embryos that are homozygous for mutated Rb genes can still develop to term.
C Development of retinoblastoma during childhood is always fatal.
D Proto-oncogenes are only expressed in damaged cells.
E The p53 gene prevents neoplasia.

(Answers overleaf)

5.1 **A** **False** The association is with squamous cell carcinoma.
    B **True** There is a weak link. There is a much stronger link between *H. pylori* and MALT (mucosa-associated lymphoid tissue) lymphoma of the stomach.
    C **False** There is a strong link with both.
    D **False** They are associated with hepatocellular adenoma.
    E **False** Therefore UV light is significantly less carcinogenic.

5.2 **A** **True** Like HIV it is an RNA retrovirus which integrates with the host using reverse transcriptase.
    B **True** Epstein–Barr virus and hepatitis B virus are also DNA viruses.
    C **True** It is thought that its main effect is immunosuppression and associated neoplasms are caused by other factors.
    D **True** It is also associated with Burkitt's lymphoma.
    E **False** EBV and malaria infection are cofactors.

5.3 **A** **True**
    B **False** It is converted in the liver to 1-hydroxy-2-naphthylamine which only becomes unconjugated and therefore active in the urinary tract.
    C **True** It is also a risk factor in bladder tumours.
    D **True** They become active by being hydroxylated.
    E **False** They alkylate DNA. Some chemotherapeutic drugs work in the same way, e.g. cyclophosphamide.

5.4 **A** **False** It is an anti-oncogene or tumour suppressor gene: non-functioning mutations of both genes leads to tumour formation.
    B **False** It is incompatible with life.
    C **False** But there is an increased risk of developing osteosarcoma later in life.
    D **False** They function in normal cells but are under strict control. When this control is lost they promote neoplasia.
    E **True** It causes damaged cells to undergo apoptosis.

5.5 Regarding tumour types:
A Sarcomas derive from mesenchymal tissue.
B Choristomas are malignant.
C Blastomas mainly occur in children.
D Benign melanomas do not occur in humans.
E Teratomas are more sensitive to radiotherapy and chemotherapy than are carcinomas.

5.6 Regarding metastasis:
A 'Pagetoid' spread refers to horizontal spread through the epithelium.
B Ocular melanomas preferentially metastasize to the brain.
C Bony metastases from prostate carcinoma are most commonly found in the pelvic and lumbar spine.
D Bony metastases from breast carcinoma are most commonly found in the shoulder girdle.
E Bony metastases from breast carcinoma cause increased bone formation.

5.7 Breast carcinoma:
A Is more common in the obese.
B Has a worse prognosis if it is oestrogen receptor-positive than if it is oestrogen receptor-negative.
C Is more common with late menarche.
D Is more common with late menopause.
E Whether oestrogen receptor-positive or oestrogen receptor-negative, responds to treatment with tamoxifen.

5.8 Regarding screening:
A It should have high levels of sensitivity and specificity.
B Highly specific tests will have high true negativity rates.
C The only aim for screening is to reduce mortality.
D Faecal occult blood is a reliable screening method for people with a strong family history of colorectal carcinoma.
E Women undergoing mammography for screening always have two views taken.

5.9 Regarding staging and grading:
A The grade of a tumour describes its extent of growth.
B Low-grade tumours have a worse prognosis than high-grade tumours.
C Manchester staging applies to breast carcinoma.
D Dukes' stage B includes lymph node involvement.
E Clark staging of melanoma involves defining invasion of different anatomical levels.

(Answers overleaf)

5.5	A	True	Carcinomas derive from epithelial tissue.
	B	False	They are benign growths of mature tissue in an ectopic site.
	C	True	They derive from embryonal cells, e.g. nephroblastoma (Wilms' tumour).
	D	True	
	E	True	This gives them a relatively good prognosis even if metastatic.

5.6	A	True	This is commonly seen in melanomas.
	B	False	They spread to the liver.
	C	True	
	D	False	They are found in the thoracic vertebrae.
	E	False	They secrete parathyroid hormone-related peptide to increase bone resorption.

5.7	A	True	There is a link between a diet high in saturated fats and carcinoma of the breast.
	B	False	The prognosis is better.
	C	False	It is more common with early menarche.
	D	True	This is due to longer exposure to oestrogens.
	E	True	

5.8	A	True	
	B	True	They will also have a low false positive rate.
	C	False	It should also reduce morbidity.
	D	False	Sensitivity and specificity are poor, so colonoscopy is more widely used.
	E	False	Two views are taken on first presentation but subsequently only one is required.

5.9	A	False	It describes the potential for growth.
	B	False	High-grade tumours progress more rapidly.
	C	True	
	D	False	The tumour breaches the muscularis propria only.
	E	True	Breslow staging involves measuring the maximum invasive depth.

6. Immunology

6.1 Regarding the complement system:
A   It is part of the specific immune response.
B   The alternative pathway is triggered by contact with exposed bacterial capsules.
C   The membrane-associated complex (MAC) is an opsonin.
D   The formation of the MAC is catalysed by C5-convertase.
E   C3b and C4b are opsonins.

6.2 Regarding antibodies:
A   Upon first exposure to an antigen, B cells will produce IgM.
B   IgG has four subclasses.
C   IgA deficiency predisposes to mucosal infections.
D   Antibodies tend to recognize antigens that are conformational (folded into a three-dimensional shape).
E   IgM is a pentameric antibody.

6.3 Of the autoimmune diseases:
A   All are disorders of the specific immune response.
B   HLA-B27 is associated with ankylosing spondylitis and anterior uveitis.
C   There is a major histocompatibility complex (MHC) association with Graves' disease.
D   They are more common in men.
E   Systemic lupus erythematosus (SLE) is characterized by antimitochondrial antibodies.

6.4 Regarding transplantation and rejection:
A   Organ transplantation requires ABO matching.
B   Human leukocyte antigen (HLA) matching is not always required in transplantation.
C   20% of allogeneic renal grafts are lost annually after the first year.
D   Acute rejection occurs within 5 days.
E   Hyperacute rejection is caused by pre-existing antibodies which fix complement.

(Answers overleaf)

6.1	A	False	It has no specificity and so is part of the innate defence.
	B	True	The classical pathway requires antigen–antibody complexes.
	C	False	It inserts into bacterial cell membranes enabling them to be lysed.
	D	True	C5-convertase is formed by the cleavage of C3 by C3-convertase.
	E	True	

6.2	A	True	Class-switching to another antibody requires T cell help.
	B	True	They are IgG1 to IgG4 which have different Fc regions and therefore different properties.
	C	True	IgA is found predominantly on mucosal surfaces and prevents adherence and penetration by pathogens.
	D	True	T cells tend to recognize linear epitopes.
	E	True	

6.3	A	True	
	B	True	
	C	True	It is associated with DR3.
	D	False	They are more common in women.
	E	False	It is characterized by antinuclear antibodies.

6.4	A	True	
	B	True	Matching may be impractical because of time constraints, e.g. in heart transplants. Also, organs in immunoprivileged sites will not need matching, e.g. the cornea.
	C	False	It is 3–5% that are lost.
	D	False	Accelerated rejection occurs within 5 days, acute rejection within a few weeks only.
	E	True	The phase occurs within minutes or hours.

6.5   In organ transplantation:
A   Graft-versus-host disease is mediated by B cells.
B   Graft-versus-host disease can occur in small bowel transplantation.
C   Kidneys are transplanted into the intraperitoneal right iliac fossa.
D   Cardiac transplants have a 5-year survival of 90%.
E   Immunosuppression for renal transplants should begin during surgery.

6.6   Regarding tumour immunology:
A   CA125 is a cytokine secreted by adenocarcinomas.
B   Beta human chorionic gonadotrophin (β-HCG) is raised in testicular tumours.
C   Non-viral lymphoid tumours have an increased incidence in the immunosuppressed.
D   Tumours can avoid the immune system by reducing human leukocyte antigen (HLA) expression.
E   Human T lymphotrophic virus 1 (HTLV-1) causes Burkitt's lymphoma.

6.7   Regarding the immune response:
A   The spleen is important for antibody production, particularly IgG.
B   Burns injuries activate the complement pathway.
C   Following surgery there is secondary immunodeficiency.
D   Perioperative blood transfusions may have an immunosuppressive effect.
E   Immunological impairment is caused by splenectomy.

6.8   Regarding immunodeficiency:
A   Chronic granulomatous disease (CGD) is caused by a neutrophil deficiency.
B   CGD is an X-linked disease.
C   Premature children have low IgG levels.
D   Regular vaccinations help delay symptoms in primary antibody deficiency (PAD).
E   Patients with severe combined immunodeficiency (SCID) will require a bone marrow transplant for survival before reaching adulthood.

6.9   Corticosteroids:
A   Reduce B cell levels.
B   Increase T cell levels.
C   Act synergistically with cyclosporin.
D   Can cause cataracts.
E   Can cause diabetes.

(Answers overleaf)

6.5   **A**   **False**   T lymphocytes in donor tissue can attack the host. This is most commonly seen in bone marrow transplantation.
      B   **True**   This is due to Peyer's patches and mesenteric lymph nodes containing large numbers of T cells.
      C   **False**   They are extraperitoneal.
      D   **False**   The survival is 75%.
      E   **False**   It should begin 4–12 hours pretransplantation.

6.6   **A**   **False**   It is a cell surface antigen.
      B   **True**   Alpha-fetoprotein is also raised in non-seminomas.
      C   **True**   Viral-induced B cell lymphomas are also more common.
      D   **True**
      E   **False**   HTLV-1 causes T cell leukaemia; Epstein–Barr virus (EBV) causes Burkitt's lymphoma.

6.7   **A**   **False**   It mainly produces IgM.
      B   **True**   They do this via the alternative pathway.
      C   **True**   Infection is often caused by breaching the gut mucosal barrier and translocation of phagocytes. This is facilitated by haemorrhagic shock, ischaemia and gut immobility. The presence of drains or other foreign bodies also provides both a route of entry and a nidus of infection.
      D   **True**   Blood transfusion should be minimized where possible.
      E   **True**   The spleen is a major site of antibody production (particularly IgM) and a reservoir of lymphocytes. Splenectomy results in a T cell lymphocytosis and an impaired antibody response to the polysaccharide antigens of bacterial capsules.

6.8   **A**   **True**   Patients present in childhood with numerous abscesses.
      B   **True**   Although an autosomal form does exist.
      C   **True**   Maternal IgG transfer predominates in the last few weeks of pregnancy.
      D   **False**   As the patient cannot produce antibodies vaccination is useless.
      E   **True**

6.9   **A**   **True**   They promote apoptosis.
      B   **False**   They inhibit proliferation and cytokine secretion.
      C   **True**
      D   **True**
      E   **True**

6.10   Of the immunosuppressive drugs:

   A   Azathioprine is selectively immunosuppressive.

   B   Hair loss is a side-effect of azathioprine.

   C   Cyclosporin is selectively immunosuppressive.

   D   Cyclosporin A derives from a fungus.

   E   Cyclosporin causes gingival atrophy.

(Answers overleaf)

6.10 **A** **False** It acts indiscriminately on all cells of the immune system.
   B **True** This is due to the effect of the drug on cells with a high proliferative rate.
   C **True** It is T cell specific.
   D **True** It is lipid-soluble.
   E **False** It can cause gingival hyperplasia as well as being nephrotoxic and hepatotoxic.

7. Basic microbiology

7.1 Regarding Gram-negative anaerobes:
A Klebsiella is normally found in the human intestine.
B Children are routinely vaccinated against *Haemophilus influenzae* type A.
C Campylobacter is the most common cause of bacterial food poisoning in the UK.
D Salmonella infection can cause osteomyelitis.
E *H. influenzae* does not constitute part of the body's normal flora.

7.2 Regarding Gram-positive bacteria:
A They stain pink in Gram staining.
B *Streptococcus faecalis* is classified as Lancefield group A.
C *Strep. faecalis* is sensitive to cephalosporins.
D *Clostridium difficile* causes gas gangrene.
E *Strep. pneumoniae* consists of diplococci.

7.3 The following antibiotics potentiate warfarin:
A Metronidazole.
B Ciprofloxacin.
C Gentamicin.
D Erythromycin.
E Trimethoprim.

7.4 Regarding penicillins and cephalosporins:
A Penicillin V is used for surgical prophylaxis in rheumatic heart disease.
B Augmentin contains a potassium salt.
C Clavulanic acid has no significant antibacterial activity.
D Cephradine is a third-generation cephalosporin.
E Cefuroxime is active against pseudomonas.

7.5 Regarding other antibiotics:
A Erythromycin belongs to the quinolone group of antibiotics.
B Methicillin-resistant *Staphylococcus aureus* (MRSA) is only sensitive to vancomycin.
C A common side-effect with oral erythromycin is constipation.
D Gentamicin can be used in pregnancy if levels are regularly monitored.
E Gentamicin is active against anaerobes.

(Answers overleaf)

7.1 A **True** It is a common cause of urinary tract infections.
 B **False** They are vaccinated against type B *H. influenzae*.
 C **True**
 D **True**
 E **False** It can be found in the respiratory tract.

7.2 A **False** Gram-negative bacteria stain pink; Gram-positive stain blue.
 B **False** It is Lancefield group D.
 C **False** It is resistant to cephalosporins but sensitive to ampicillin.
 D **False** *C. perfringens* (or *welchii*) causes gas gangrene. *C. difficile* causes pseudomembranous colitis.
 E **True** It can cause pneumonia, bronchitis and meningitis.

7.3 A **True**
 B **True**
 C **False**
 D **True**
 E **True** It also potentiates phenytoin.

7.4 A **True** It is also used following splenectomy.
 B **True** It consists of amoxycillin and potassium clavulanate.
 C **True** It inhibits β-lactamase thereby rendering penicillinase-producing bacteria sensitive to amoxycillin.
 D **False** It is first generation.
 E **False** Second-generation cephalosporins are not active against pseudomonas but third-generation cephalosporins are.

7.5 A **False** Erythromycin is a macrolide. Ciprofloxacin is an example of a quinolone.
 B **False** Teicoplanin is chemically related to vancomycin and is also active against MRSA.
 C **False** It commonly causes diarrhoea.
 D **False** It is contraindicated because of nephrotoxicity and ototoxicity.
 E **False** It is active against staphylococci and coliforms.

7.6   Regarding skin infections and abscesses:
A   Breast abscesses are most commonly caused by *Staphylococcus epidermidis*.
B   Abscesses can spread via the bloodstream.
C   A furuncle is an infection of a hair follicle.
D   Erysipelas is caused by *Streptococcus pyogenes*.
E   Necrotizing fasciitis is initially treated with high-dose antibiotics.

7.7   Regarding clostridial infections:
A   *C. perfringens* is normally found in the bowel.
B   *C. tetani* is an aerobic Gram-positive bacillus.
C   The neurotoxin produced by *C. tetani* activates the spinal reflexes, thereby causing spasm.
D   Loss of consciousness is not a feature of tetanus.
E   Tetanus does not have an incubation period.

7.8   Regarding transmissible infections:
A   Screening for methicillin-resistant *Staphylococcus aureus* (MRSA) should include swabs from the axilla.
B   After treatment of MRSA, swabs should be checked at 3 days and 7 days.
C   An operation on a wound involving a human bite is classified as contaminated.
D   Shaving the operation site should take place immediately before surgery.
E   Nosocomial infections occur in about 10% of patients.

7.9   Regarding HIV and hepatitis:
A   HIV-positive patients should be placed last on an operating list.
B   Staff suffering from needlestick injuries with HIV-positive blood should immediately have chemoprophylaxis with zidovudine.
C   Hepatitis B cannot be transmitted by droplets.
D   The incubation period of hepatitis B virus is between 4 days and 4 weeks.
E   Hepatitis C is not associated with carcinoma of the liver.

(Answers overleaf)

7.6 **A** **False** The most common cause is *Staph. aureus.*
     B **True** An example of a 'metastatic' abscess is infective endocarditis causing cerebral abscesses.
     C **True** It is commonly known as a boil.
     D **True** It responds well to penicillin.
     E **False** Wide excision of necrotic tissue along with antibiotics is imperative.

7.7 **A** **True**
     B **False** It is anaerobic.
     C **False** The toxin blocks the inhibitory activity at the spinal reflexes, thereby causing spasm.
     D **True** The patient remains conscious throughout the convulsions.
     E **False** The incubation period is 1–30 days.

7.8 **A** **True** Swabs should also be taken from the perineum, groin, hairline and nose.
     B **False** They should be checked at 3 days and 3 weeks later.
     C **True** Open fractures and operations involving opening the colon are also classified as contaminated.
     D **True** This reduces the chance of infection particularly by staphylococci.
     E **True**

7.9 **A** **False** This will make their operations more likely to be cancelled.
     B **False** There is no clear evidence that zidovudine works and side-effects are common: nausea, vomiting and headache.
     C **False**
     D **False** It is between 6 weeks and 6 months.
     E **False**

7.10   In severe infection:

A   Temperature below 36°C is one of the criteria for defining SIRS (systemic inflammatory response syndrome).

B   In the development of SIRS, stage II is when cytokines are released into the local environment.

C   The two main interleukins involved in SIRS and MODS (multiple organ dysfunction syndrome) are IL-1 and IL-6.

D   Prognosis in multi-organ failure is about 50% survival with one organ affected.

E   Septicaemia following burns is commonly due to *Staphylococcus aureus*.

(Answers overleaf)

7.10 **A** **True**   Other criteria are:
- temperature > 38°C
- heart rate > 90 b.p.m.
- respiratory rate > 20/min
- $PaCO_2$ < 4.3 kPa
- WBC > 12 000 cells/mm^3
- WBC < 4000 cells/mm^3
- or 10% immature forms.

     B **False** This is stage I. Stage II is when cytokines are released into the circulation.

     C **True**

     D **False** Prognosis is 70% survival with one organ affected, 50% survival with two organs affected.

     E **True**   Coliforms and bacteroides are also implicated.

8. Nervous system

8.1   Regarding the meninges:
A   The falx cerebri lies between the two cerebral hemispheres.
B   The free border of the tentorium cerebelli surrounds the pons.
C   The subdural space contains the cerebral arteries.
D   The subarachnoid space extends up to the level of the L2 vertebra only.
E   Blood vessels entering the ventricles carry a sleeve of pia mater.

8.2   Regarding the dural venous sinuses:
A   They have more valves than do veins of similar size.
B   The transverse sinus continues as the internal jugular vein.
C   The cavernous sinus is closely related to the pituitary gland.
D   The cavernous sinus has all three divisions of the trigeminal nerve on its lateral wall.
E   Facial infection can spread to the cavernous sinus through the pterygoid plexus.

8.3   Complete transection of the oculomotor nerve results in:
A   Ptosis.
B   Convergent squint.
C   Constriction of pupil.
D   Loss of accommodation and light reflex.
E   Diplopia.

8.4   Regarding the facial nerve:
A   It emerges through the stylomastoid foramen.
B   It lies deep to the parotid gland.
C   The mandibular branch is related to the submandibular gland.
D   If the upper part of the face is spared, the lesion is above the pons.
E   The greater petrosal nerve is one of its branches.

(Answers overleaf)

8.1 **A** **True** Anteriorly the falx is attached to the crista galli and posteriorly to the tentorium cerebelli.

B **False** The free border forming the tentorial notch surrounds the midbrain. The cerebral peduncles (part of the midbrain), oculomotor nerves and posterior cerebral arteries are all related to this and may be involved in a transtentorial herniation.

C **False** Most cerebral vessels are in the subarachnoid space. The subdural space is traversed by veins draining into the dural venous sinuses.

D **False** The spinal cord extends up to the upper border of L2 in the adult. The meninges, the dural sheath and the subarachnoid space extend up to the level of S2.

E **True** These form the tela choroidea of the choroid plexus.

8.2 **A** **False** The sinuses are valveless.

B **False** It continues as the sigmoid sinus which becomes the internal jugular vein.

C **True** The gland lies medial to the cavernous sinus.

D **False** It has the oculomotor, trochlear, ophthalmic and maxillary division of the trigeminal on the lateral wall. The internal carotid artery and the abducens nerve are more medial.

E **True** The facial vein is connected to the pterygoid plexus which in turn is connected to the cavernous sinus by emissary veins.

8.3 **A** **True** It is due to paralysis of levator palpebrae superioris.

B **False** There is divergent squint due to unopposed action of lateral rectus and superior oblique.

C **False** The constrictor pupillae is paralysed and hence the pupil is dilated.

D **True** This is due to paralysis of ciliary muscles and constrictor pupillae.

E **True** It is due to paralysis of extraocular muscles.

8.4 **A** **True** The nerve then enters the parotid gland.

B **False** It lies within the substance of the gland superficial to the retromandibular vein and the external carotid artery.

C **True** It lies below the lower border of the mandible and is vulnerable in incisions in this region.

D **True** This will be a supranuclear paralysis (upper motor neuron). The nucleus lies in the pons.

E **True** This and the chorda tympani branch are given off as the nerve passes through the canal in the temporal bone.

8.5   Regarding the sympathetic nervous system:
A   The stellate ganglion is related to the vertebral artery.
B   The thoracic ganglia are related to the posterior intercostal arteries.
C   The left lumbar sympathetic ganglia lie behind the abdominal aorta.
D   Removal of first thoracic ganglion causes Horner's syndrome.
E   Removal of lumbar sympathetics may compromise ejaculation.

8.6   Regarding control of cerebral blood flow (CBF):
A   CBF is mainly regulated by the sympathetic nervous system.
B   Cerebral arterioles constrict when the blood pressure increases.
C   CBF remains constant in the blood pressure range between 50–150 mmHg.
D   Hypocapnia increases CBF.
E   CBF remains constant over a wide range of PaO_2.

8.7   Regarding cerebrospinal fluid (CSF):
A   It is produced in the lateral, III and IV ventricles.
B   It enters the subarachnoid space through the foramina of Luschka and Magendie.
C   It is reabsorbed mostly into the lymphatics.
D   Its rate of production is mostly dependent on the CSF pressure.
E   It can be sampled from the cisterna magna.

(Answers overleaf)

8.5 **A** **True** The ganglion lies on the neck of the first rib and the transverse process of the seventh cervical vertebra and is related anteriorly to the vertebral and the subclavian arteries.

B **True** The thoracic part of the trunk lies on the heads of the ribs behind the costal pleura and descends in front of the intercostal vessels.

C **True** The right chain is overlapped anteriorly by the inferior vena cava.

D **True** The syndrome is characterized by ptosis, miosis and anhydrosis on the side of the lesion.

E **True** Parasympathetic stimulation causes erection and the sympathetics are involved in ejaculation.

8.6 **A** **False** Neural factors are relatively less important in the regulation of CBF. Regulation is achieved mostly by myogenic and metabolic factors.

B **True** This is part of the myogenic regulation of CBF. The vessels constrict as the blood pressure increases and dilate as the pressure drops.

C **True** CBF is remarkably constant within this blood pressure range.

D **False** Hypocapnia causes vasoconstriction and a reduction in CBF; hyperventilation causing hypocapnia is used to treat raised intracranial pressure by reducing CBF.

E **True** Vascular responses to PaO_2 are not as marked as those induced by changes in $PaCO_2$.

8.7 **A** **True** CSF is produced in the choroid plexuses of the lateral, III and IV ventricles. From the lateral ventricle it flows into the III ventricle through the interventricular foramen (Munro) and then though the cerebral aqueduct into the IV ventricle.

B **True** The foramina of Luschka and Magendie are seen on the roof of the IV ventricle.

C **False** CSF is reabsorbed mostly through arachnoid villi and granulations into the dural venous sinuses. About 15% is absorbed in the lumbar area in villi similar to arachnoid villi or along the nerve sheaths into the lymphatics.

D **False** The rate of production is relatively independent of blood pressure and CSF pressure (normal being 120–180 mmH$_2$O). The rate of absorption depends on the CSF pressure.

E **True** But samples are usually withdrawn from the lumbar cistern by doing a lumbar puncture.

8.8   The blood–brain barrier:
A   Is produced by a thin layer of collagen between the blood vessels and the nervous tissue.
B   Is permeable at birth.
C   Is usually permeable to glucose and hydrogen ions.
D   Is absent in the posterior pituitary.
E   Is absent in the area postrema.

8.9   Regarding pain relief:
A   Stimulation of large sensory fibres transmitting heat or pressure may inhibit smaller pain fibres.
B   There are descending fibres in the spinal cord which are involved in pain relief.
C   NSAIDs relieve pain by inhibiting prostaglandins.
D   Opioid peptides are derived from the juice of the opium poppy.
E   Opioids are most effective when injected intravenously.

8.10   To certify brain stem death the following reflexes are tested:
A   Light reflex.
B   Corneal reflex.
C   Accommodation reflex.
D   Gag reflex.
E   Vestibulo-ocular reflex.

(Answers overleaf)

8.8 **A** **False** It is produced by the tight junctions between endothelial cells and the end-feet processes of astrocytes.

B **True** The barrier is permeable at birth as evidenced by the passage of bilirubin into the nervous system when its blood level is markedly raised.

C **False** It is permeable to glucose and fat-soluble drugs. Hydrogen ion crosses the barrier only in chronic acidic conditions. The barrier maintains a constant interstitial environment around the neurons, which are sensitive to alterations in ionic concentrations.

D **True** Antidiuretic hormone and oxytocin pass directly into the bloodstream. It is also absent in the median eminence of the hypothalamus where the releasing and inhibitory hormones pass into the capillaries.

E **True** This is related to the vomiting centre and is sensitive to morphine, digoxin, creatinine and ketone bodies.

8.9 **A** **True** Impulses of large fibres inhibit cells in the substantia gelatinosa shutting the 'gate' to the ascent of impulses from the smaller pain fibres.

B **True** These lie in the dorsolateral funiculus of the spinal cord and exert control over pain input. They may also release endorphins and enkephalins.

C **True** Prostaglandins stimulate the release of inflammatory agents such as histamine and bradykinin, which in turn stimulate nociceptors.

D **False** Opiates are drugs derived from the opium poppy. Opioids are non-opiate compounds which bind to the opiate receptors.

E **False** They are endogenous analgesic peptides binding to opioid receptors.

8.10 **A** **True** Both direct and consensual light reflexes should be absent.

B **True** There should be no response to direct stimulation of the cornea.

C **False** The patient is deeply unconscious.

D **True** There should be no gagging when the back of the throat is touched with a catheter.

E **True** There should be no eye movement following slow injection of 50 ml of cold water over a minute into each external auditory meatus in turn. This tests cranial nerves VIII, III and VI.

8.11 Regarding intracranial haemorrhage:
    A Extradural haemorrhage may be associated with fracture of the temporal bone.
    B In an extradural haemorrhage a lucid interval may be followed by brain stem compression.
    C Subdural haematoma is always caused by severe head injury.
    D Subarachnoid haemorrhage may have a non-traumatic cause.
    E Subarachnoid haemorrhage often is not fatal.

8.12 Transtentorial herniation causes:
    A Ipsilateral pupillary dilatation.
    B Contralateral hemiparesis.
    C Ipsilateral hemiparesis.
    D Cortical blindness.
    E Hydrocephalus.

8.13 Regarding cerebral tumours:
    A All astrocytomas are benign and occur in childhood.
    B Medulloblastoma occurs in early middle age.
    C Glioblastoma multiforme is malignant.
    D Meningiomas arise from the dura mater.
    E Acoustic neuroma shows cerebellar signs and raises the intracranial pressure relatively early.

(Answers overleaf)

8.11 **A** **True**   Injury is often to the middle meningeal artery following a fracture of the temporal bone. The haematoma lies outside the dura and causes brain compression.

 B **True**   A lucid interval occurs when the clot is organized. This is followed by increase in intracranial pressure which may lead to transtentorial herniation and brain stem compression.

 C **False**   Acute subdural haemorrhage follows head injury. However, chronic subdural haemorrhage occurring in the elderly is due to brain shrinkage making the bridging veins (between the cerebral cortex and the dural venous sinuses) in the subdural space vulnerable to trivial head injury.

 D **True**   It can often be due to rupture of a 'berry' aneurysm. It can also be caused by hypertension, coagulation disorders, rupture of a vascular malformation, tumours and vasculitis.

 E **True**   15% of cases are instantly fatal, a further 45% dying later because of rebleeding.

8.12 **A** **True**   It is due to oculomotor nerve paralysis.

 B **True**   It is due to compression of the ipsilateral cerebral peduncle.

 C **True**   It is due to compression of the contralateral cerebral peduncle.

 D **True**   It is due to compression of the posterior cerebral artery.

 E **True**   It is due to compression of the cerebral aqueduct.

8.13 **A** **False**   They vary in malignancy and the peak incidence is in early middle age. In children, the tumour is benign, occurs often in the cerebellum and may show cystic changes.

 B **False**   This is the commonest glioma in childhood. It arises in the roof of the IV ventricle and infiltrates into the cerebellum. It may cause obstructive hydrocephalus.

 C **True**   This is the most malignant brain tumour and occurs between 40–60 years.

 D **False**   Meningiomas arise from arachnoid cells. They are usually benign and prognosis after excision is good.

 E **False**   These signs rarely occur. Sensorineural deafness with tinnitus is a common manifestation. There may be facial nerve involvement at a later stage. Loss of corneal reflex, dysphagia and dysarthria are other signs produced by involvement of cranial nerves.

8.14   Regarding spinal cord injuries and compression:
  A   The anal and bulbocavernous reflexes are the first to return after spinal shock.
  B   Anterior cord lesion is characterized by loss of touch and proprioception below the level of the lesion.
  C   Central cord syndrome may be caused by a hyperextension injury.
  D   Brown–Sequard syndrome is caused by hemisection of the cord.
  E   Cauda equina syndrome is characterized by an autonomous bladder.

8.15   In peripheral nerve injury:
  A   Laceration of a nerve causes neuropraxia.
  B   Wallerian degeneration occurs in axonotmesis.
  C   In nerotmesis, axon, myelin sheath and endoneurial tube are severed.
  D   The rate of regeneration is about 1 mm per day.
  E   Best results after regeneration are in mixed nerves.

(Answers overleaf)

8.14 **A** **True** These depend on intact sacral segments and reflex arcs. The anal reflex shows contraction of the anal sphincter when the perianal skin is stimulated with a pin. The bulbocavernous reflex is contraction of the anal sphincter in response to squeezing the glans penis.

B **False** These are the characteristics of a posterior cord lesion affecting the posterior column. There will be profound ataxia due to loss of proprioception in a posterior cord syndrome, whereas in an anterior cord syndrome there is loss of muscle power and reduction of pain and temperature sensation below the level of the lesion.

C **True** This is seen in older patients with cervical spondylosis. The spinal cord is compressed between osteophytes and intervertebral disc in front and thickened ligamentum flavum behind. The more centrally situated cervical tracts supplying the arm are affected more than the peripherally placed tracts controlling the legs.

D **True** Classical signs are ipsilateral motor paralysis (pyramidal tract), loss of proprioception and touch (posterior column) and loss of pain and temperature sensation on the opposite side (spinothalamic).

E **True** Lumbosacral nerve roots are compressed causing lower motor neuron type of bladder and bowel dysfunction.

8.15 **A** **False** There is loss of conduction but no anatomical disruption in neuropraxia. Recovery is rapid and complete.

B **True** The axon is divided and degenerates distal to the site of injury. Degeneration starts about 3–4 days after injury. Regeneration occurs provided the endoneurial tube is intact.

C **True** This occurs in a nerve laceration.

D **True** An individual nerve may not regenerate into its original nerve sheath. Motor axon may grow into a sensory sheath and vice versa. The functional results may not be good.

E **False** Best results are in purely motor and purely sensory nerves or in nerves joined by surgery.

9. Cardiovascular system

9.1   During the development of the heart and great vessels:
A   The sinus venosus becomes incorporated into the right atrium.
B   The foramen ovale is the gap between the septum primum and the endocardial cushions.
C   The septum secundum develops to the right of the septum primum.
D   The fourth aortic arch becomes the subclavian artery on the left side.
E   The right recurrent laryngeal nerve hooks around the sixth aortic arch on the right side.

9.2   Regarding congenital abnormalities of the heart and great vessels:
A   Ventricular septal defects (VSDs) always require surgical repair.
B   Eisenmenger's syndrome is associated with cyanosis.
C   Patent ductus arteriosus (PDA) causes left-to-right shunt.
D   Fallot's tetralogy features a stenosed aortic outflow tract.
E   Coarctation of the aorta produces notching of the inferior borders of the ribs.

(Answers overleaf)

9.1 **A** **True** The smooth portion of the right atrium is derived from the sinus venosus.

B **False** The foramen ovale (ostium secundum) develops as a hole in the upper part of the septum primum. The gap between the septum primum and the endocardial cushions is known as the ostium primum.

C **True** During fetal life this acts like a valve allowing blood to flow from the right to the left side. At birth, rise in left atrial pressure forces the septum primum and septum secundum together. They fuse, obliterating the foramen ovale and leaving a dimple known as the fossa ovalis.

D **False** The fourth aortic arch on the left side becomes the arch of the aorta. However, on the right side it contributes to the subclavian artery.

E **False** The sixth aortic arch on the right side disappears. The fifth arch artery also disappears and the recurrent laryngeal nerve thus winds round the fourth arch (subclavian artery) on the right side. On the left, the sixth arch artery remains as the ductus arteriosus and the left recurrent laryngeal nerve hooks round it. The larynx originally developed at the level of the sixth aortic arch.

9.2 **A** **False** Small defects in the muscular part of the septum may close spontaneously. Large defects in the membranous part may require repair.

B **True** Eisenmenger's syndrome seen in the late stages of ASD (atrial septal defect), VSD or PDA is associated with right-to-left shunt and cyanosis. This is produced as a consequence of increased pulmonary flow leading to pulmonary hypertension.

C **True** The ductus arteriosus connects the left pulmonary artery to the aorta and causes left-to-right shunt until its late stage (Eisenmenger's syndrome).

D **False** The four features are pulmonary stenosis, VSD, overriding of the aorta into both the ventricles and right ventricular hypertrophy.

E **True** This feature, seen on chest X-ray, is due to enlargement of the intercostal arteries which lie along the inferior borders of ribs. Vessels around the scapula, internal mammary and epigastric arteries are also enlarged.

9.3 Regarding the chambers of the heart:
A The interatrial septum has the crista terminalis.
B The sinoatrial (SA) node is situated near the opening of the coronary sinus.
C The right atrium should be incised along its right border.
D Chordae tendineae and papillary muscles prevent mitral and tricuspid regurgitation.
E The atrioventricular (AV) bundle is the only pathway by which impulses can reach the ventricles from the atria.

9.4 Regarding the coronary arteries:
A The right coronary artery arises from the anterior aortic sinus below the aortic valve.
B The left coronary artery passes behind the pulmonary trunk.
C The right coronary artery supplies the SA node.
D The left anterior descending is a branch of the left coronary artery.
E The circumflex artery is a branch of the right coronary artery.

(Answers overleaf)

9.3 **A** **False** The crista terminalis separates the smooth part of the atrium (developed from the sinus venosus) from the rough part derived from the primitive atrium. The fossa ovalis is seen in the interatrial septum.

B **False** The SA node is situated at the upper end of the crista terminalis. The AV node is near the opening of the coronary sinus.

C **True** This is to avoid damage to the SA node.

D **True** These prevent the tricuspid and mitral valve cusps being everted back into the atria during ventricular systole.

E **True** The fibrous skeleton at the atrioventricular junction is electrically inert. The only structure through which impulses can pass across this is the AV bundle.

9.4 **A** **False** The coronary sinuses are just above the aortic valves on the ascending aorta. The right coronary artery arises from the anterior sinus and the left from the left aortic sinus.

B **True** It then lies between the pulmonary trunk and the left auricle before reaching the atrioventricular groove.

C **True** In 60% of the population the right coronary supplies the SA node; in the remaining 40% it is supplied by the circumflex branch of the left coronary artery. The AV node is supplied by the posterior interventricular (posterior descending) branch of the right coronary artery in 90% of the population.

D **True** This artery, also known as the 'widow maker', is much larger than the posterior descending artery. It runs down to the apex of the heart in the atrioventricular groove and gives off the diagonal arteries.

E **False** The circumflex, a branch of the left coronary artery, winds round the left surface of the heart to anastomose with the branches of the right coronary. It may be large ('left dominance') in about 10% of the population giving off the posterior interventricular branch.

9.5   Regarding the descending thoracic aorta:

A   It extends from the lower border of the fourth thoracic vertebra to the lower border of the twelfth.

B   The oesophagus lies on its right side throughout.

C   The hemiazygos veins are behind.

D   The thoracic duct is in close contact on its left side.

E   Operations on thoracic aneurysms may interfere with the blood supply of the spinal cord.

9.6   The abdominal aorta:

A   Is related anteriorly to the third part of the duodenum but is separated from it by the pancreas.

B   Has the right renal vein in a posterior relation.

C   Is at risk when inserting a needle into the abdomen to obtain a pneumoperitoneum in a slim person.

D   Has the inferior vena cava closely applied to its right side.

E   Has the inferior mesenteric vein running close to it on the left side.

(Answers overleaf)

9.5 **A** **True** It is the continuation of the arch of the aorta. The upper part lies on the left surface of the vertebra, the lower end is in the midline.

B **False** The oesophagus is on its right side in the upper part. But as it descends it crosses in front of the aorta to lie on its left side in the lower part.

C **True** The left intercostal veins drain into these and they in turn drain into the azygos vein.

D **False** The thoracic duct lies on the right side of the descending aorta.

E **True** Radicular arteries, branches of the posterior intercostal arteries from the descending aorta, reinforce the spinal arteries. They are known as the 'booster' or 'feeder' vessels. The largest is known as the arteria radicularis magna (of Adamkiewicz) which most commonly is at 10th or 11th thoracic level, but the level of origin is prone to variation.

9.6 **A** **False** The third part of the duodenum crosses it anteriorly. The head of the pancreas is above the duodenum. An inflammatory aneurysm may be adherent to the third part of the duodenum and an anastomosis between a graft and the aorta at this level has a risk of developing a fistula into the duodenum causing haematemesis and melaena.

B **False** The left renal vein crosses the aorta anteriorly just below the origin of the superior mesenteric artery. An aneurysm at this level may stretch the vein markedly. The vein may have to be divided; this is done as far to the right as possible to preserve its tributaries, i.e. gonadal and adrenal veins, which can act as venous collaterals.

C **True** The lumbar vertebrae with their large bodies and forward convexity can make the abdominal aorta and the inferior vena cava close to the anterior abdominal wall.

D **True** It gradually becomes more posterior at its lower end. The iliac veins lie behind the iliac arteries.

E **True** The vein is close to the aorta at the level of the renal vessels and may be damaged during resection of an aneurysm, especially if it is associated with a large haematoma.

9.7   Regarding the common femoral artery:
A   It divides into superficial and deep femoral.
B   Pulsation can easily be felt at the midinguinal point.
C   The profunda femoris arises from its medial aspect.
D   It lies medial to the femoral vein.
E   The inguinal lymph nodes are closely applied to its walls.

9.8   The popliteal artery:
A   Extends from the adductor hiatus to the lower border of the popliteus muscle.
B   Lies superficial to the popliteal vein.
C   Has the tibial nerve lateral to it throughout.
D   May be exposed by an incision along the course of the great saphenous vein.
E   Has the tibioperoneal trunk as a branch.

9.9   Regarding the right subclavian artery:
A   It is closely related to the pleura at the apex of the right lung.
B   The right vagus nerve crosses its posterior surface.
C   The second part lies in front of the scalenus anterior.
D   The lower trunk of the brachial plexus lies behind the artery.
E   The first part normally has no branches.

(Answers overleaf)

9.7 **A** **True** The deep femoral is also known as the profunda femoris, the superficial femoral being the continuation of the main artery into the adductor canal.

 B **True** This is a convenient site for taking arterial samples for blood gases and for insertion of catheters.

 C **False** The profunda femoris or deep femoral artery arises on the lateral side and just below its origin is crossed by a branch from the profunda vein. Ligation and division of the vein exposes the profunda femoris artery.

 D **False** The vein lies medial to the artery.

 E **False** The superficial inguinal nodes lie along the great saphenous vein and the inguinal ligament. The deep nodes are in the femoral canal medial to the femoral vein. In a block dissection of the groin the superficial and deep fascia, the saphenous vein and the fatty and lymphatic content of the femoral triangle are removed leaving only the femoral artery, vein and nerve.

9.8 **A** **True** The adductor hiatus can be exposed above the knee by incising the fascia on the roof of the adductor canal after an incision along the medial border of the sartorius.

 B **False** The artery lies deep to the vein.

 C **False** The nerve crosses from lateral to medial.

 D **True** This is deepened to expose the medial border of the medial head of the gastrocnemius, which is retracted to expose the artery.

 E **True** The other terminal branch is the anterior tibial. The tibioperoneal trunk, which is surrounded by a venous plexus, is 2 cm long and bifurcates into the posterior tibial and peroneal arteries.

9.9 **A** **True** The pleura is separated by the suprapleural membrane.

 B **False** The vagus crosses in front of the artery at its medial end where it gives off the right recurrent laryngeal nerve which loops under the artery, travelling posteromedially, to reach the groove between the trachea and oesophagus.

 C **False** The second part of the artery lies behind the scalenus anterior muscle. In surgical exposure of the artery, the muscle is divided after retracting the phrenic nerve on its surface medially.

 D **True** The lower trunk is formed by the nerve roots C8 and T1.

 E **False** The first part has three branches, the vertebral artery, the thyrocervical trunk and the internal thoracic artery.

9.10   The long (great) saphenous vein:
A   Lies 1–2 cm anterior to the medial malleolus.
B   Passes a hand's breadth behind the lateral border of the patella.
C   Joins the femoral vein 3–4 cm inferolateral to the pubic tubercle.
D   Has the saphenous nerve closely applied to it at the knee.
E   Contains more valves below the level of the knee than above.

9.11   Regarding cardiac contraction:
A   It is caused by the binding of calcium ions to troponin C.
B   The y descent of the venous pulse is caused by the atrium relaxing and the tricuspid valve moving down during early systole.
C   At no moment are all four heart valves closed at the same time.
D   The ejection fraction is the stroke volume divided by the left ventricular end-diastolic volume.
E   The sinoatrial (SA) node and conducting system do not have a resting membrane potential.

9.12   Regarding the coronary circulation:
A   The conducting system is more commonly supplied by the right coronary artery.
B   Coronary blood flow tends to occur in systole.
C   The heart uses carbohydrates more than fats as an energy source.
D   Oxygen consumption from the blood is minimal during rest leaving a large reserve for exercise.
E   Autonomic innervation is of most importance in regulating coronary vessel tone.

9.13   Regarding blood pressure:
A   Mean pressure is calculated by adding half the pulse pressure to the diastolic pressure.
B   Baroreceptors are found in the walls of the atria.
C   Renin is released when there is a decrease in kidney perfusion.
D   Transection of the spinal cord above the thoracolumbar region causes spinal shock.
E   The Hagen–Poiseuille law states that flow in a tube is inversely related to the length of the tube.

(Answers overleaf)

9.10 **A** **True** This is a constant position which can be used for a cut-down in an emergency.

B **False** It passes a hand's breadth behind the medial border of the patella.

C **True** It passes through the saphenous opening piercing the cribriform fascia to reach the femoral vein. The long saphenous vein has a number of tributaries at this level.

D **False** The nerve is closely applied to it in the lower calf. The vein is usually stripped only to just below the knee to avoid damage to the nerve.

E **True**

9.11 **A** **True** Calcium ions are released from the sarcoplasmic reticulum by the arrival of the action potential.

B **False** This is the cause of the x descent. The y descent is caused by the tricuspid valve opening and blood flowing during diastole.

C **False** They are all closed during isovolumetric contraction when the volume remains constant but pressure increases.

D **True** It is approximately 60%.

E **True** They are constantly depolarizing and repolarizing.

9.12 **A** **True**

B **False** It occurs during diastole as the intramyocardial vessels are compressed during systole.

C **False** Energy derivation is 60% from fats, 35% from carbohydrates, and 5% from ketones.

D **False** Oxygen consumption is near maximal at rest. Flow must increase to provide more oxygen.

E **False** Local metabolites, e.g. potassium and adenosine, are much more important.

9.13 **A** **False** It is one-third of the pulse pressure plus diastolic pressure.

B **False** They are located in the carotid sinus and the aorta.

C **True** Renin acts on angiotensinogen to produce angiotensin I which converts to angiotensin II – a vasopressor.

D **True** It is due to a loss of sympathetic vasomotor tone.

E **True** The whole equation is:

$$\text{Flow} = \frac{P\pi r^4}{8\eta l}$$

where P = pressure; r = radius; η = viscosity; l = length.

9.14   Regarding shock:
A   Septic shock leads to vasodilatation.
B   Hartmann's solution will be of benefit in hypovolaemic shock.
C   The body can maintain blood pressure until 50% of the circulation is lost.
D   Aerobic metabolism provides 36 moles of ATP for each mole of glucose.
E   Septic patients will hypoventilate to prevent alkalosis.

9.15   In cardiac monitoring:
A   The P–R interval is < 0.12 seconds.
B   The normal pulmonary capillary wedge pressure is 15–20 mmHg.
C   During continuous monitoring of the blood pressure, the area under the waveform is proportional to the stroke volume.
D   Cardiac output can be measured using a temperature dilution technique using warm glucose solution.
E   Circulating bilirubin gives falsely low readings on the pulse oximeter.

9.16   Regarding cardiac support:
A   Nitrates reduce both afterload and preload.
B   Noradrenaline's main effect is on β-receptors.
C   Adrenaline has both α and β effects.
D   Adrenaline causes renal vasodilatation.
E   A 'renal dose' of dopamine is approximately 10 μg/kg/min and will not stimulate the heart.

9.17   In atherosclerosis:
A   Fatty streaks contain a proliferation of smooth muscle cells.
B   Gelatinous plaques commonly occur in small arteries.
C   The fibro-fatty plaque causes thickening of the tunica media.
D   Even small fibro-fatty plaques cause narrowing of the lumen.
E   Plaque may undergo calcification.

(Answers overleaf)

9.14 **A** **True** A similar picture is seen in high transection of the spinal cord.

B **True** However, it will pass into both circulatory and interstitial spaces, so colloids are initially preferable.

C **False** Losses greater than 20% cause falls in blood pressure and cardiac output.

D **True** Anaerobic metabolism provides only 2 moles of ATP for each mole of glucose.

E **False** They hyperventilate in response to acidosis due to lactic acid build-up.

9.15 **A** **False** The P–R interval should be between 0.12–0.21 seconds.

B **False** It is 6–12 mmHg. Higher pressures will cause pulmonary oedema.

C **True** The up-slope is proportional to the myocardial contractility.

D **False** The glucose used is cold.

E **True** Carboxyhaemoglobin, on the other hand, gives falsely high readings.

9.16 **A** **True** They do this by reducing total peripheral resistance and venodilatation.

B **False** It mainly acts on α_1 receptors.

C **True**

D **False** It causes vasoconstriction and can lead to acute renal failure.

E **False** Doses greater than 4 µg/kg/min will begin to increase the heart rate and contractility.

9.17 **A** **False** Proliferation of smooth muscle cells occurs in fibro-fatty plaques. It is not a feature of fatty streaks.

B **False** They are usually seen in the aorta and large arteries.

C **False** The intima is thicker than the media. Medial thinning by the plaque leads to aneurysm.

D **False** Narrowing does not occur until the plaques are quite thick. Coronary plaques must occupy at least 40% of the arterial wall before they can be detected radiologically.

E **True** This may be patchy or extensive.

9.18   The following are major risk factors in atherosclerosis:
A   Cigarette smoking.
B   Hypocholesterolaemia.
C   Hypertension.
D   Diabetes insipidus.
E   Age.

9.19   In atherosclerosis:
A   Shear stress and turbulence are causative factors.
B   There is increased lipid absorption into the intima.
C   Low-density lipoprotein (LDL) is oxidized by free radicals at the site of endothelial injury.
D   Intimal thickening is mainly due to proliferation of collagen.
E   Platelet-derived growth factor (PDGF) promotes smooth muscle cell proliferation.

9.20   Regarding platelets:
A   They are derived from macrophages.
B   They adhere to normal endothelial cells.
C   Platelet activating factor is the major stimulus for platelet activation.
D   Aspirin prevents platelet adhesion.
E   Primary aggregation is larger than secondary aggregation.

(Answers overleaf)

9.18 **A** **True** Smoking causes endothelial changes, reduction of prostaglandins, increased level of low-density lipoprotein (LDL), and platelet aggregation.

B **False** Hypercholesterolaemia is a major risk factor. Lowering the cholesterol level with statins has shown considerable benefits, especially in secondary prevention.

C **True** It is a major risk factor at all ages. It seems that it is the increased level of blood pressure that causes the damage. In coarctation of the aorta, atherosclerosis develops in high-pressure vessels proximal to the stenosis, but not distally where the pressure is low.

D **False** Diabetes mellitus is a major risk factor. Diabetics have higher levels of LDL and triglycerides and lower levels of high-density lipoprotein (HDL).

E **True** The risk of myocardial infarction and stroke increases with each decade right up to advanced age.

9.19 **A** **True** These mechanical factors exaggerate the effects of other causative factors such as hypertension.

B **True** Intimal permeability is increased by endothelial injury resulting in increased absorption of lipids.

C **True** Oxidized LDL is toxic to endothelial cells and attracts monocytes and macrophages.

D **False** Smooth muscle cells from the tunica media migrate into the intima and they proliferate to increase the thickness of the intima at the expense of the media.

E **True** PDGF, produced by platelets, endothelial cells and macrophages, is a stimulant for smooth muscle cell proliferation.

9.20 **A** **False** They are derived from megakaryocytes. Each megakaryocyte produces about 3000 platelets as they circulate in the lung.

B **False** Platelet accumulation and adhesion follows endothelial injury.

C **False** It is only one of many factors, others being thrombin, collagen, trypsin and thromboxane.

D **True** Aspirin (and even alcohol in moderate quantities) inhibits thromboxane production by inhibiting the cyclo-oxygenase pathway of arachidonic acid metabolism.

E **False** In secondary aggregation the aggregates are larger and are associated with secretion from the platelets.

9.21   Regarding ischaemic heart disease:
A   The inner third of the heart muscle is better perfused than the outer third.
B   The anterior descending branch of the left coronary is frequently involved.
C   Depression of the ST segment is the hallmark of cardiac ischaemia.
D   Papillary muscle infarct and pericarditis may complicate a transmural infarct.
E   The time interval between the onset of ischaemia and irreversible changes is about 24 hours.

9.22   Regarding valvular heart disease:
A   Mitral stenosis causes left ventricular hypertrophy.
B   Mitral regurgitation is occasionally a feature of Marfan's syndrome.
C   Aortic stenosis can occur because of calcification of the valve.
D   Ankylosing spondylitis may be associated with aortic regurgitation.
E   Thromboembolism is more likely with bioprosthesis than with mechanical valves.

9.23   Reperfusion injury may cause:
A   Compartment syndrome.
B   Hypokalaemia and acidosis.
C   Myoglobinaemia.
D   Pulmonary oedema.
E   Gastrointestinal changes.

9.24   Abdominal aortic aneurysms:
A   Are more common in males than in females.
B   Are associated with thinning of the intimal layer of the vessel.
C   Rarely contain mural thrombus.
D   May occlude the renal arteries.
E   Often rupture when the diameter is greater than 60 mm.

(Answers overleaf)

9.21 **A** **False** The inner third is the least well perfused and is the site of a subendocardial infarct.

 B **True** Approximately 50% of infarcts affect this branch.

 C **True** The degree of depression of the ST segment is a rough indication of the severity of the myocardial injury.

 D **True** Rupture of papillary muscle produces severe regurgitation and cardiac failure.

 E **False** The time interval is much shorter, about 12 hours, during which period fibrinolysis and/or angioplasty may help.

9.22 **A** **False** It gradually causes left atrial hypertrophy, and then pulmonary oedema with brown induration of the lung.

 B **True** Aortic regurgitation may also occur.

 C **True** This usually happens in old age.

 D **True** It occurs as a consequence of aortic root dilatation.

 E **False** It is more likely with mechanical valves and patients require long-term anticoagulation treatment.

9.23 **A** **True** It is a result of swelling in fascial compartments.

 B **False** There may be hyperkalaemia due to leakage of potassium from damaged cells and acidosis due to build-up of acidic metabolites.

 C **True** It is due to breakdown of muscle cells, and can result in acute tubular necrosis.

 D **True** It is due to increased permeability of pulmonary vasculature and sequestration of neutrophils.

 E **True** There is gastrointestinal oedema which may lead to increased GI vascular permeability and endotoxic shock.

9.24 **A** **True** The incidence in men is about five times higher than in women.

 B **False** The media is atrophied and the elastic fibres are replaced by collagen.

 C **False** Mural thrombus is common and may fill the saccular aneurysm.

 D **True** They may occlude the iliac vessels also.

 E **True** About 80% die of rupture, if left untreated.

9.25 Dissecting aneurysms:
A Most commonly affect the popliteal artery.
B Have a peak incidence in the third decade of life.
C Are confined to the intima.
D May be associated with Marfan's syndrome.
E May cause myocardial infarction (MI).

9.26 Regarding varicose veins:
A They are more common in women.
B The saphenofemoral junction is initially affected.
C Haemosiderin deposition causes pigmentation.
D High venous pressure causes lipodermatosclerosis.
E There is a higher incidence of venous thrombosis in those who take oral contraceptives.

(Answers overleaf)

9.25 **A** **False** They most commonly affect the thoracic aorta.
      B **False** The elderly are most affected.
      C **False** They may start as a tear in the intima and then the dissection extends to affect most of the media.
      D **True** But all patients with the syndrome may not have this.
      E **True** When the ascending aorta is affected, it may dissect across the coronary ostium leading to MI or it may dissect across the aortic valve causing aortic regurgitation.

9.26 **A** **False** But women consult their doctors about them more often.
      B **True** As the vein stretches, the lower valves will be affected progressively.
      C **True**
      D **True** The high venous pressure distends the capillaries and facilitates deposition of fibrin and other materials. Diffusion of oxygen and nutrients to the tissue is reduced leading to necrosis, sclerosis and ulceration.
      E **True** There is a strong association with the oestrogen content of the pill.

10. Haemopoietic and lymphoreticular system

10.1 **Erythrocytes:**
A   Live for up to 6 months.
B   Require vitamin B_{12} for their production (erythropoiesis).
C   Are produced in red marrow found in the humerus and femur in adults.
D   Are produced by a process of meiosis and maturation.
E   Make haemoglobin in their immature, reticulocyte, stage.

10.2 **Regarding anaemias:**
A   Red cell life span is reduced in haemolytic anaemias.
B   Priapism is associated with sickle cell disease.
C   In HbS, valine is replaced by glutamic acid.
D   Hereditary spherocytosis is due to a defect in haemoglobin.
E   MCV (mean cell volume) is calculated by dividing red cell concentration by haematocrit.

10.3 **Regarding white blood cells:**
A   The half-life of neutrophils in the blood is 2–3 days.
B   Neutropenia is the most common form of leukopenia.
C   Neutrophils and eosinophils are functionally similar.
D   Eosinophils are involved in the allergic response.
E   Basophils release histamine.

10.4 **Regarding haemostasis:**
A   Von Willebrand's disease is an X-linked recessive disorder.
B   Haemophilia A is due to a lack of factor IX.
C   Platelet counts less than $100 \times 10^9/l$ will lead to spontaneous bleeding.
D   Plasmin converts fibrinogen to fibrin.
E   There is increased fibrinogen in disseminated intravascular coagulation (DIC).

10.5 **Regarding anticoagulation:**
A   Cimetidine potentiates the action of warfarin.
B   Heparin potentiates the action of antithrombin III.
C   Factor X is common to both intrinsic and extrinsic pathways.
D   Alopecia is a long-term side-effect of heparin.
E   Warfarin affects the intrinsic system.

(Answers overleaf)

10.1 **A** **False** They survive for 18–120 days.
      B **True** Iron and folate are also needed.
      C **True** Other sites in the adult are skull, ribs and axial skeleton.
      D **False** Cells divide by mitosis.
      E **True** Reticulocytes contain RNA and ribosomes before maturing into erythrocytes.

10.2 **A** **True** Blood films will show sickled cells, spherocytes and red cell fragments.
      B **True**
      C **False** Glutamic acid cannot be coded for and so is replaced by valine.
      D **False** The defect is in the red cell membrane.
      E **True** The range is 78–98 fl.

10.3 **A** **False** It is only 6–12 hours.
      B **True** Counts less than 0.5×10^9/l can lead to sepsis.
      C **False** Neutrophils and monocytes both phagocytose and digest foreign material.
      D **True** Increased levels are also seen in parasitic infections.
      E **True** They are functionally similar to tissue mast cells.

10.4 **A** **False** It is autosomal dominant.
      B **False** It is due to lack of factor XIII. Haemophilia B is due to factor IX deficiency.
      C **False** Counts usually have to be less than 20×10^9/l for spontaneous bleeding to occur.
      D **False** Thrombin converts fibrinogen to fibrin. Plasmin converts fibrin to fibrin degradation products (FDP).
      E **False** There are decreased platelets, decreased fibrinogen and increased FDPs in DIC.

10.5 **A** **True** It inhibits breakdown by the liver.
      B **True**
      C **True** Working along with factor V and calcium, it converts prothrombin to thrombin.
      D **True** Other side-effects are osteoporosis and thrombocytopenia.
      E **False** Warfarin affects the extrinsic system. Heparin affects the intrinsic system.

10.6 Regarding the lymphatic system:
A Antigen is presented to B cells via T helper cells in the cortex of lymph nodes.
B T cells are predominantly found in the paracortex of lymph nodes.
C Blockage of lymphatics causes fat malabsorption.
D The thoracic duct drains into the right subclavian vein.
E Milroy's disease presents at puberty.

10.7 Regarding the anatomy of the spleen:
A The splenic artery is a branch of the hepatic artery.
B The spleen has a cortex and medulla.
C The white pulp mainly contains T lymphocytes.
D The spleen is attached to the left kidney by peritoneum.
E The splenic vein and inferior mesenteric vein join to form the portal vein.

10.8 Regarding splenic dysfunction:
A After splenectomy, the red cell count is raised.
B After splenectomy, the platelet count is raised.
C Splenomegaly may be seen in infectious mononucleosis.
D Pneumococcal vaccine should be given after splenectomy.
E Mitral valve defects can affect the spleen.

10.9 Regarding the thymus:
A It does not have a capsule.
B Thymic tumours commonly metastasize.
C It develops from the second pharyngeal pouch.
D Its blood supply is from the internal mammary artery.
E It is at its largest at puberty.

10.10 Regarding blood cells:
A Platelets survive in the circulation for up to 30 days.
B Packed cell volume and total blood volume are both raised in polycythaemia.
C Erythrocytes are removed from the circulation by macrophages.
D Reticulocytes remain in the circulation for 7–10 days before maturing to erythrocytes.
E The globin part of the erythrocyte is converted into bilirubin.

(Answers overleaf)

10.6 **A** **True**
    B **True** They are mainly helper/inducer cells.
    C **True** Lymph flow is aided by peristalsis of the vessel wall.
    D **False** It drains into the left subclavian vein.
    E **False** It is congenital lymphoedema and presents at birth.

10.7 **A** **False** It is a branch of the coeliac trunk.
    B **False** Lymph nodes have a cortex and medulla. The spleen has red and white pulp.
    C **False** It mainly contains B lymphocytes. The red pulp has a predominance of red blood cells.
    D **True** The lienorenal ligament envelopes the tail of the pancreas and splenic vessels.
    E **False** The splenic vein and superior mesenteric vein form the portal vein.

10.8 **A** **False** It remains the same but Howell–Jolly bodies may be seen.
    B **True**
    C **True** It may also be seen in malaria and typhoid.
    D **False** It should be given before splenectomy because residual splenic function contributes to the immune response.
    E **False** Tricuspid valve incompetence can lead to increased pressure in the inferior vena cava which is transmitted to the spleen via the portal vein.

10.9 **A** **False** The capsule extends into the thymus as trabeculae, dividing it into lobules.
    B **False** Metastases are very rare.
    C **False** It develops from the third and fourth pharyngeal pouches.
    D **True** Alternatively, it is from the pericardiophrenic arteries.
    E **True**

10.10 **A** **False** They survive for 8–10 days.
    B **True**
    C **True** This occurs in the spleen.
    D **False** They mature in 1–2 days.
    E **False** The haem part forms bilirubin; the globin releases amino acids.

11. Respiratory system

11.1 The trachea is situated in close relation to:
A   The isthmus of the thyroid gland.
B   The right subclavian artery.
C   The left recurrent laryngeal nerve, not the right.
D   The carotid sheath.
E   The thoracic duct.

11.2 Regarding the bronchi and bronchopulmonary segments:
A   The left main bronchus gives off the upper lobe bronchus just before it enters the lung.
B   The left main bronchus crosses the oesophagus and the descending aorta.
C   The right main bronchus lies in front of the pulmonary artery.
D   Each bronchopulmonary segment is ventilated by a terminal bronchiole.
E   Each lung has 10 bronchopulmonary segments.

11.3 Regarding the pleura:
A   The cervical pleura extends 2.5 cm above the lateral aspect of the clavicle.
B   A needle passed through the fourth and fifth intercostal spaces immediately lateral to the sternum on the right side will enter the pericardium without passing through the pleural cavity.
C   It descends below the medial end of the 11th rib but not the 12th.
D   The parietal pleura is sensitive only to stretching.
E   Inflammation of the pleura can present as abdominal pain.

(Answers overleaf)

11.1 **A** **True** The thyroid isthmus is adherent to tracheal rings 2, 3 and 4.

B **False** On the right side the brachiocephalic artery is closely related to the thoracic part of the trachea. The right subclavian branches off from it but is more lateral.

C **False** Both the recurrent laryngeal nerves lie in the groove between the trachea and oesophagus in the neck.

D **True** The carotid sheath is a close relation to the cervical part of the trachea laterally, also the lateral lobes of the thyroid gland.

E **False** The thoracic duct is closely related to the oesophagus, not the trachea. The azygos vein is related to the lower part of the trachea on the right side and hooks over the right bronchus to join the superior vena cava.

11.2 **A** **False** The left bronchus divides inside the lung, whereas the right gives off its upper lobe branch just outside the lung.

B **True** It is an anterior relation of the oesophagus and the descending aorta.

C **False** The artery is first below and then anterior to the bronchus. Bronchus lies posterior to the pulmonary vessels at the root of the lung on both sides.

D **False** Branches of the lobar bronchi (i.e. tertiary bronchi) ventilate the bronchopulmonary segments. Terminal bronchioles are of very small diameters and are the generation of bronchioles just proximal to the respiratory bronchioles.

E **True** Each is supplied by a segmental bronchus, artery and vein. Each segment is functionally independent and takes its name from that of the supplying segmental bronchus.

11.3 **A** **False** At the sternal end of the clavicle the pleura rises 2.5 cm above it.

B **False** This is true on the left side as the pleura deviates more laterally at these levels, whereas on the right side it extends up to the midline.

C **False** It descends below the medial end of the 12th rib and can be inadvertently opened during exposure of the kidney or adrenal gland.

D **False** It is supplied by somatic nerves and is sensitive to pain. The visceral pleura is sensitive only to stretch as it is supplied by the autonomic nerves.

E **True** The costal pleura is supplied by the intercostal nerves which also supply the anterior abdominal wall to which the pain can be referred.

11.4   Regarding the diaphragm:
A   It is attached to the lower six ribs.
B   The aortic orifice transmits the left vagus nerve along with the aorta.
C   The oesophageal orifice lies in the left crus.
D   The inferior vena caval opening lies in the central tendon.
E   Damage to the phrenic nerve results in elevation of the diaphragm on the paralysed side.

11.5   In the superior mediastinum:
A   The trachea divides at the upper border of T4.
B   The arch of the aorta gives off three of its major branches.
C   The thoracic duct is related to the oesophagus.
D   The remnant of the thymus is present posteriorly.
E   The superior vena cava is formed by the union of the two brachiocephalic veins.

11.6   Regarding chemoreceptors:
A   They increase their firing rate in response to increased pH.
B   Peripheral chemoreceptors are solely found in the carotid bodies.
C   Increased arterial $PaCO_2$ causes cerebral vasodilatation.
D   Hydrogen ions easily cross the blood–brain barrier.
E   Cerebrospinal fluid (CSF) has a lower buffering capacity than blood.

11.7   Regarding compliance and resistance:
A   Compliance decreases on lying supine.
B   Compliance decreases in emphysema.
C   Prematurity is a risk factor for atelectasis.
D   Smaller alveoli have lower pressures according to the law of Laplace.
E   Sympathetic nerves cause bronchodilatation.

(Answers overleaf)

11.4 **A** **True** Attachment is to their inner aspects, and it continues on to the xiphoid process.

B **False** The aortic orifice transmits the azygos vein and the thoracic duct besides the aorta. The vagus nerves (gastric nerves) enter the abdomen along with the oesophagus.

C **False** The orifice is surrounded by the fibres of the right crus.

D **True** It also transmits the right phrenic nerve.

E **True** It also shows paradoxical movement due to pressure difference in the abdomen and thorax.

11.5 **A** **False** The trachea divides at the level of the lower border of T4; the superior mediastinum is above the plane connecting the sternal angle to the lower border of T4.

B **True** They are the brachiocephalic artery, the left common carotid and the left subclavian.

C **True** It lies along the left border of the oesophagus.

D **False** The remnant of the thymus is anterior.

E **True** The superior vena cava is joined by the azygos vein at the level of the sternal angle.

11.6 **A** **False** They increase their firing rate in response to decreased pH, decreased PaO_2 and increased $PaCO_2$.

B **False** They can also be found in the aortic arch.

C **True**

D **False** CSF hydrogen ion content changes in response to CO_2 concentration.

E **True** However, HCO_3^- can diffuse slowly in the CSF, thereby buffering CO_2 increases and 'resetting' the chemoreceptors, e.g. in chronic obstructive pulmonary disease (COPD).

11.7 **A** **True**

B **False** Compliance also increases with age.

C **True** This is due to a lack of surfactant which reduces surface tension.

D **False** They have greater pressures. Laplace's law states that the pressure in a bubble is equal to twice the wall tension divided by the radius.

E **True**

11.8 Regarding respiratory function tests:
A Physiological dead space includes the anatomical dead space.
B Closing capacity increases with age.
C Functional residual capacity cannot be measured by spirometry.
D Anatomical dead space increases on standing.
E The FEV_1/FVC ratio is increased in pulmonary fibrosis.

11.9 Regarding blood gases:
A The liver is the main organ responsible for compensatory changes to respiratory acidosis/alkalosis.
B Mixed venous blood has an oxygen tension of 8 kPa.
C Metabolic acidosis is associated with hyperkalaemia.
D 2,3-diphosphoglyceric acid (DPG) comes mainly from leukocytes.
E A rise in temperature shifts the oxyhaemoglobin dissociation curve to the right.

11.10 Regarding hypoxaemia and its causes:
A Hypoxaemia due to a shunt is significantly improved by administering supplemental oxygen.
B Hypoxaemia due to diffusion impairment is not significantly improved by administering supplemental oxygen.
C In hypoventilation, $PaCO_2$ increases much more than PaO_2 decreases.
D Ventilation–perfusion ratio increases from base to apex.
E Arterial $PaCO_2$ is normally raised in shunts.

11.11 With regard to oxygenation:
A Transfer factor relates to the transfer of oxygen and carbon dioxide in the peripheral tissues.
B Haemoglobin has a greater affinity for carbon monoxide than for oxygen.
C Carbon monoxide shifts the oxyhaemoglobin dissociation curve to the left.
D Oxygen saturation in normal mixed venous blood is 75%.
E HbS results in a shift of the dissociation curve to the left.

11.12 Positive pressure ventilation:
A Increases dead space.
B Can cause pneumothorax.
C Increases venous return.
D Can cause hypocapnoea.
E In the form of IPPV (intermittent positive pressure ventilation) maintains positive pressure at the end of expiration.

(Answers overleaf)

11.8 **A** **True**   Physiological dead space includes the anatomical dead space and the alveolar dead space.

      B **True**   This is the volume of the lungs when the small airways start to close.

      C **True**   Nitrogen washout, helium dilution or body plethysmography is required.

      D **True**

      E **True**   FVC decreases more than FEV_1.

11.9 **A** **False**   The kidney is the principal organ for regulating H^+ and HCO_3^- excretion.

      B **False**   It is only 5.3 kPa.

      C **True**   There is increased uptake of H^+ ions in exchange for K^+ ions by the cells.

      D **False**   It is found in red blood cells.

      E **True**   As also does a fall in pH and an increase in $PaCO_2$ and 2,3-DPG.

11.10 **A** **False**   Because of the flat top of the oxyhaemoglobin dissociation curve, alveolar oxygen content rises little.

      B **False**   Diffusion is proportional to the oxygen concentration gradient.

      C **True**   If alveolar ventilation is halved, $PaCO_2$ is doubled.

      D **True**   The apices are much more poorly ventilated than the bases.

      E **False**   Chemoreceptors ensure a rise in ventilation if $PaCO_2$ rises.

11.11 **A** **False**   It relates to the diffusion capacity of the lung.

      B **True**

      C **True**   This causes decreased unloading of oxygen at specific oxygen tensions.

      D **True**

      E **False**   The curve is shifted to the right.

11.12 **A** **True**   Higher airways pressure causes blood to be diverted away from ventilated regions.

      B **True**

      C **False**   Therefore cardiac output should be measured and inotropic support considered.

      D **True**   It is due to hyperventilation.

      E **False**   This is PEEP (positive end expiratory pressure).

11.13 Regarding respiratory failure:
A Hypercapnia causes headache and papilloedema.
B In chronic respiratory failure with raised $PaCO_2$ the body adapts to a consistently low pH.
C Lack of oxygen supply to the brain can be tolerated for 3 minutes.
D Hypercapnia occurs when $PaCO_2$ rises above 8.5 kPa.
E Lactic acidosis occurs as a response to hypercapnia.

11.14 In adult respiratory distress syndrome:
A Chest X-ray shows diffuse shadowing.
B There is ventilation–perfusion mismatch.
C Lung compliance increases.
D Fat embolism is a cause.
E PEEP (positive end expiratory pressure) can be useful.

11.15 The posterior mediastinum:
A Extends inferiorly from level T2.
B Contains the splanchnic nerves.
C Contains the hemiazygos vein.
D Contains the thymus.
E Terminates at the level of the 10th thoracic vertebra.

11.16 Regarding lung infections:
A Lobar pneumonia commonly occurs in the early postoperative period.
B *Streptococcus pneumoniae* and *Haemophilus influenzae* are causative organisms.
C Red 'hepatization' is a feature of bronchopneumonia.
D Lobar pneumonia may mimic appendicitis.
E Aspiration pneumonia may be caused during anaesthesia.

11.17 Adult respiratory distress syndrome:
A Can occur in patients with multi-system trauma.
B Is associated with shock.
C Is characterized by a reduction in pulmonary compliance.
D Is contributed by endothelial damage and free radical production is seen.
E Is followed by full recovery in most cases.

(Answers overleaf)

11.13 **A** **True** They are due to an increased cerebral blood flow.
 B **False** pH is not much lower than normal owing to retention of bicarbonate by the kidneys.
 C **True** After 3 minutes irreversible changes occur.
 D **False** A level above 6.5 kPa is considered to be raised.
 E **False** Hypoxia causes a switch from aerobic to anaerobic metabolism.

11.14 **A** **True**
 B **True** It is due to poorly ventilated units.
 C **False** There is alveolar collapse and oedema.
 D **True** Other causes are sepsis, burns and chest trauma.
 E **True** It helps by decreasing alveolar oedema and increasing ventilation.

11.15 **A** **False** It extends downwards from the horizontal plane through the sternal angle at the level of T4.
 B **True**
 C **True**
 D **False** This lies in the superior mediastinum.
 E **False** It terminates at T12.

11.16 **A** **False** Bronchopneumonia is more common; it is due to failure of removal of respiratory tract secretions.
 B **True** These are the common organisms; *Staphylococcus aureus* and coliforms are rarer. *Staph. aureus* pneumonia is seen in hospital patients after influenza and also in drug abusers.
 C **False** Red hepatization occurs in lobar pneumonia about 24 hours after its onset. The lung is red, solid and airless and resembles the cut surface of fresh liver.
 D **True** It does so by causing referred pain in the abdomen.
 E **True** It can occur during induction and/or recovery.

11.17 **A** **True** It can also occur after direct lung trauma.
 B **True** It is associated with shock due to any cause.
 C **True** There is diffuse alveolar damage with hyaline membranes.
 D **True** There is also alveolar damage and loss of surfactant.
 E **False** About 50% die despite intensive therapy.

11.18 Regarding primary carcinoma of the lung:

    A   Metastasis is through the lymphatics and blood.

    B   The 5-year survival rate is about 30%.

    C   Oat cell carcinomas are amenable to surgical resection.

    D   Squamous cell carcinomas are situated in the periphery of the lung.

    E   Adenocarcinomas are associated with asbestosis.

(Answers overleaf)

11.18 A   True   This happens quickly. Only about 15% are operable at
                      diagnosis.

    B   False   5-year survival is only about 5%.

    C   False   They are widely invasive, metastasize early and are not
                      resectable. The first line of treatment is chemotherapy.

    D   False   They arise centrally in a major bronchus; adenocarcinoma
                      tends to occur in the periphery.

    E   True   Exposure to asbestos also causes mesothelioma of the
                      pleura.

12. Locomotor system

12.1 Regarding the lumbar vertebrae:
  A   The vertebral body has large foramina for basivertebral veins.
  B   They do not allow rotary movements.
  C   The spinal cord ends at the level of the upper border of the first lumbar vertebra.
  D   The highest point of the iliac crest is at the level of the gap between L3–L4 spines.
  E   L5 nerve root passes into the L5–S1 intervertebral foramen.

12.2 Regarding the intervertebral disc:
  A   Its superior and inferior surfaces are lined with fibrocartilage.
  B   The posterior longitudinal ligament is firmly attached to it.
  C   The nucleus pulposus is in the centre.
  D   The nucleus pulposus usually herniates anteriorly.
  E   It is avascular throughout life.

12.3 The vertebral canal:
  A   Does not extend below L1 in the adult.
  B   Contains the anterior longitudinal ligament.
  C   Is bounded anterolaterally by the vertebral laminae.
  D   Is bounded by the pedicles.
  E   Contains the vertebral venous plexus.

(Answers overleaf)

12.1 **A** **True** The basivertebral veins are valveless and malignant tumours can metastasize into the bone through these veins.

B **True** Rotation is mostly at the thoracic level.

C **False** The cord ends at its lower border, the meninges and the CSF extend further down into the sacral canal.

D **True**

E **True** Each lumbar nerve comes out below the corresponding lumbar vertebra.

12.2 **A** **False** Hyaline cartilage lines the surfaces.

B **True** However, the posterior longitudinal ligament is not firmly attached to the vertebral bodies, allowing the basivertebral veins to emerge from them.

C **False** The nucleus pulposus is more towards the posterior aspect of the disc than at its centre. It is surrounded by the fibrocartilaginous annulus fibrosus which has collagen fibres in concentric laminae, each lamina perpendicular to the adjacent one.

D **False** It usually herniates posterolaterally and may press on the nerve roots.

E **False** It is mostly avascular after childhood. The periphery of the disc (which is mostly collagen) has few vessels. Nutrients reach the disc by diffusion from the vertebral bodies.

12.3 **A** **False** The vertebral canal continues into the sacrum as the sacral canal.

B **False** The anterior longitudinal ligament lies on the anterior surface of the vertebrae.

C **True** Laminae are linked by ligamenta flava. Anteriorly, the vertebral canal is bounded by the bodies of the vertebrae, intervertebral discs and the posterior longitudinal ligament.

D **True** The intervertebral foramen is bounded above and below by the pedicles, anteriorly by the intervertebral disc and posteriorly by the zygapophyseal joint.

E **True** It also contains the spinal cord, the cauda equina, the meninges and laterally the spinal nerve roots and the dorsal root ganglia.

12.4   With regard to fracture of the clavicle:
A   It fractures mostly at its medial end.
B   The costoclavicular ligament is ruptured.
C   Fracture of the outer third may rupture the coracoclavicular ligament.
D   It produces marked displacement of the bone ends.
E   The brachial plexus is often injured.

12.5   In a patient with a fracture of the surgical neck of the humerus:
A   The capsule of the shoulder joint will almost certainly be torn.
B   The nerve most likely to be damaged is the axillary nerve.
C   The brachialis muscle will probably be torn.
D   A muscle likely to be paralysed is the deltoid.
E   The proximal fragment may be abducted slightly by the deltoid.

12.6   The lateral cord of the brachial plexus:
A   Contains motor fibres only.
B   Gives rise to the musculocutaneous nerve.
C   May contribute to the ulnar nerve.
D   May be damaged in fractures of the surgical neck of the humerus.
E   Contains T1 fibres.

12.7   Regarding Erb's palsy:
A   C5 and C6 are affected.
B   Deltoid, supraspinatus, infraspinatus and teres minor are affected.
C   Triceps is paralysed.
D   The forearm is supinated.
E   It causes Horner's syndrome.

(Answers overleaf)

12.4 **A** **False** It fractures in between the two strong ligaments on either end. The usual site is the middle of the shaft of the clavicle.

B **False** This ligament is attached to the medial end of the clavicle and is not affected.

C **True** The coracoclavicular ligament is attached to the lateral end and may be ruptured. The acromioclavicular joint also may be affected.

D **False** The strong ligaments and other soft tissue attached prevent marked displacement.

E **False** Though closely related to the clavicle the subclavian vessels and brachial plexus escape injury as the displacement is minimal.

12.5 **A** **False** The fracture can be extracapsular.

B **True** The axillary nerve winds round the surgical neck of the humerus.

C **False** The muscle takes origin from the shaft below the surgical neck.

D **True** Deltoid is supplied by the axillary nerve.

E **False** Deltoid insertion is distal to the surgical neck; the distal fragment may be abducted by the deltoid.

12.6 **A** **False** All cords are mixed nerves.

B **True** The nerve branches off early, leaves the axillary sheath at a higher level and hence escapes in a brachial plexus block in the axilla.

C **True** C7 fibres in the ulnar nerve are derived from the lateral cord.

D **False** It lies on the anterolateral aspect of the axillary artery and is not related directly to the surgical neck.

E **False** It is formed by the anterior divisions of the upper and middle trunks and hence contains C5, C6, and C7 fibres and not T1.

12.7 **A** **True** It is a traction injury of the upper trunk of the brachial plexus caused by an increase in the angle between the neck and shoulder, as happens as a result of traction during shoulder presentation in childbirth or because of a fall on the point of the shoulder.

B **True** The arm will be adducted and medially rotated.

C **False** Triceps is supplied by C7 and C8. Biceps, brachialis and brachioradialis will be paralysed (C5 and C6).

D **False** Paralysis of biceps causes pronation.

E **False** T1 is not affected and hence there is no Horner's syndrome.

12.8   Regarding Klumpke's palsy:
   A   C8 and T1 roots are affected.
   B   Interossei and lumbrical muscles of the hand are paralysed.
   C   Metacarpophalangeal (MCP) and interphalangeal (IP) joints are flexed.
   D   Sensory loss will be along the lateral border of the limb.
   E   It may cause Horner's syndrome.

12.9   Regarding the radial nerve:
   A   It is the only nerve of the posterior cord which reaches the forearm.
   B   It will result in paralysis of the triceps if damaged in the middle of the arm.
   C   It runs part of its course in a groove between the brachioradialis and the brachialis.
   D   It occasionally supplies the brachialis.
   E   Paralysis produces loss of sensation along the lateral border of the forearm.

12.10 Entrapment of the posterior interosseous nerve (deep branch of the radial) as it passes through the supinator may cause:
   A   Paralysis of all the extensors of the wrist.
   B   Inability to extend the fingers at the metacarpophalangeal (MCP) joints.
   C   Paralysis of the supinator muscle.
   D   Inability to extend the interphalangeal (IP) joint of the thumb.
   E   Loss of cutaneous sensation on the dorsal surface of the thumb.

(Answers overleaf)

12.8 A True Damage is caused by excessive and violent abduction of the shoulder as may occur in a difficult breach delivery.

B True All the intrinsic muscles of the hand are affected as they are supplied by T1.

C False Interossei and lumbricals flex the MCP joints and when they are paralysed the MCP joints are extended by the unopposed extensor digitorum. The IP joints remain flexed by the long flexors because the interossei and lumbricals normally act as their antagonists at these joints.

D False Upper segments of the brachial plexus (C5, C6) supply the lateral border and the lower segments (C8, T1) the medial border.

E True Most of the sympathetic input into the head and neck is through T1.

12.9 A True The other branches of the posterior cord are the axillary nerve, thoracodorsal (to the latissimus dorsi) and subscapular nerves.

B False The long and medial heads are supplied by branches given off in the axilla.

C True After it pierces the lateral intermuscular septum it lies in front of the lateral epicondyle where it can be blocked.

D True

E False The forearm is supplied by the medial and lateral cutaneous nerves of the forearm. Radial nerve paralysis or paralysis of its superficial branch produces sensory loss that is limited to the first web space on the dorsum of the hand.

12.10 A False Extensor carpi radialis longus is supplied by the trunk of the radial nerve along with the brachioradialis.

B True This is due to paralysis of the extensor digitorum.

C False The muscle gets a branch just before the posterior interosseous pierces it.

D True The extensor pollicis longus is paralysed.

E False The deep branch has no cutaneous distribution.

12.11 Regarding the shoulder joint:
A   Stability depends mainly on the glenoid labrum.
B   The subscapularis bursa communicates with the synovial cavity.
C   The long head of triceps passes though the synovial cavity.
D   The subacromial bursa lies above the supraspinatus tendon.
E   Osteomyelitis may cause septic arthritis.

12.12 The following structures are encountered in an anterior approach for the exposure of the shoulder joint:
A   Cephalic vein.
B   Short head of biceps.
C   Subscapularis.
D   Musculocutaneous nerve.
E   Radial nerve.

12.13 Dislocation of the shoulder joint:
A   Is most commonly an anteroinferior dislocation.
B   Usually occurs as a result of a fall on the outstretched hand.
C   May damage the axillary nerve.
D   May flatten the contour of the shoulder.
E   Will cause the acromion process to be more prominent.

12.14 The following are entirely intracapsular at the elbow joint:
A   Trochlea.
B   Capitulum.
C   Medial epicondyle.
D   Lateral epicondyle.
E   Growth plates for the lower end of the humerus.

(Answers overleaf)

12.11 A False Stability depends mainly on the rotator cuff muscles, i.e. supraspinatus, infraspinatus, teres minor and subscapularis.

B True It does so through the gap in the anterior part of the capsule.

C False The long head of the biceps enclosed in a synovial sheath passes through the joint cavity.

D True The bursa separates the supraspinatus tendon from the coracoacromial ligament.

E True The capsular attachment, which is mostly to the anatomical neck, extends onto the metaphysis inferomedially. Osteomyelitis occurs in the metaphysis.

12.12 A True The vein lies in the deltopectoral groove and is encountered if the incision is along this.

B True The short head of biceps and the coracobrachialis taking origin from the coracoid process cover the anterior aspect of the shoulder. The tip of the coracoid process is detached and the two muscles retracted to expose the capsule.

C True The tendon of subscapularis, which is inserted into the lesser tubercle, reinforces the anterior aspect of the capsule. This tendon is defined and divided to expose the capsule.

D True The musculocutaneous nerve entering the coracobrachialis is vulnerable during retraction of the muscle.

E False The radial nerve from the posterior cord is given off at a lower level and is not close to the capsule of the joint.

12.13 A True The capsule is weakest in its inferior part where it is not reinforced by the rotator cuff.

B True Abduction and lateral rotation of the arm stretches the anteroinferior part.

C True The nerve passes through the quadrilateral space and is closely related to the inferior part of the joint.

D True The contour is contributed by the upper end of the humerus and the deltoid muscle.

E True This is due to displacement of the greater tubercle.

12.14 A True
B True
C False
D False
E False The growth plate for the medial epicondyle is entirely intracapsular but that for the trochlea, capitulum and lateral epicondyle is extracapsular posterolaterally.

12.15 Concerning the distal end of the radius:
A The styloid process is at a lower level compared to that of the ulna.
B It articulates distally with the scaphoid, lunate and triquetral.
C Extensor pollicis longus lies lateral to the dorsal tubercle (of Lister).
D Tendons of abductor pollicis longus and extensor pollicis brevis are related to the lateral surface.
E The distal growth plate of the radius is entirely intracapsular.

12.16 The scaphoid bone:
A Articulates with the first metacarpal bone distally.
B Is commonly fractured in the young.
C Is closely related to the tendon of the flexor carpi radialis.
D Receives its blood supply through both its proximal and distal ends.
E Has relatively less periosteum-covered area.

12.17 Regarding carpal tunnel syndrome:
A It is caused by compression of the ulnar nerve in the carpal tunnel.
B It produces wasting of the hypothenar muscles.
C It may be associated with Dupuytren's contracture.
D Pain and paraesthesia occur along the lateral aspect of the palm.
E Pressure on the nerve can be released by an incision distal to the distal skin crease of the wrist.

(Answers overleaf)

12.15 **A** **True**
  B **False** The triquetral articulates directly with the fibrocartilage between the radius and ulna.
  C **False** It is medial to the tubercle.
  D **True**
  E **False** It is entirely outside the capsule of the wrist joint.

12.16 **A** **False** It articulates with the trapezium distally, which in turn articulates with the first metacarpal bone.
  B **True** Fracture is often due to a fall on the outstretched hand.
  C **True** The tendon lies medial to the scaphoid. The scaphoid is felt in the floor of the anatomical snuff box and is also closely related to the radial artery. When fractured, there is tenderness in the anatomical snuff box.
  D **True** Sometimes the blood supply is from the distal end only, resulting in avascular necrosis of the proximal fragment when fractured.
  E **True** Hence the bone has a poor blood supply.

12.17 **A** **False** It is caused by compression of the median nerve in the carpal tunnel. The ulnar nerve passes superficial to the flexor retinaculum.
  B **False** The hypothenar muscles are supplied by the ulnar nerve. The median nerve supplies the thenar muscles. However, the flexor pollicis brevis and the opponens may also be supplied by the ulnar nerve.
  C **True** Also there is a recognized association with rheumatoid arthritis and pregnancy.
  D **False** The lateral aspect of the palm is supplied by the palmar cutaneous branch of the median nerve, which crosses superficial to the flexor retinaculum, and it is not compressed. Pain and paraesthesia are along the lateral three or four fingers, which are supplied by the median nerve in the palm.
  E **True** The tunnel is in the palm. The proximal edge of the retinaculum underlies the distal wrist crease.

12.18 Severance of the median nerve at the elbow causes:
A Paralysis of all the flexors of the fingers.
B Wasting of hypothenar muscles.
C Claw hand.
D Inability to abduct and adduct fingers.
E Sensory loss on the lateral aspect of the palm and the palmar surface of the lateral three fingers.

12.19 Severance of the ulnar nerve at the wrist causes:
A Paralysis of all the lumbricals.
B Inability to flex the terminal phalanx of the ring and little fingers.
C Sensory loss on the posterior aspect of the little finger.
D Trophic changes in the index finger.
E A positive Froment's sign.

12.20 Regarding Dupuytren's contracture:
A It is a contracture of the flexor tendons.
B The lateral aspect of the hand is affected.
C It may be hereditary.
D It may affect the foot.
E Digital nerves are vulnerable during surgery.

12.21 Regarding the pulp space:
A It contains fat and fibrous tissue.
B It contains deep flexor tendon.
C Infection causes throbbing pain.
D The periosteum of the terminal phalanx should be removed during surgery of a pulp space infection.
E Infection may lead to osteomyelitis of the whole terminal phalanx.

(Answers overleaf)

12.18 A False The medial half of the flexor digitorum profundus is supplied by the ulnar nerve.

B False The median nerve supplies the thenar muscles. Hypothenar muscles are supplied by the ulnar nerve.

C False Claw hand is caused by the loss of MCP joint flexion because of paralysis of the interossei and the lumbricals in an ulnar nerve paralysis.

D False These movements are produced by the interossei, which are supplied by the ulnar nerve.

E True These areas are supplied by the median nerve.

12.19 A False Only the medial two lumbricals are paralysed. The lateral two lumbricals are supplied by the median nerve.

B False Flexion of the distal phalanx of the little finger is done by the medial half of the flexor digitorum profundus, which is supplied by the ulnar nerve in the forearm.

C False This area is supplied by the dorsal digital branch of the ulnar nerve given off in the forearm.

D False The index finger is supplied by the median nerve.

E True This is due to paralysis of the adductor pollicis.

12.20 A False It is contracture of the palmar aponeurosis.

B False It usually affects the medial part, flexing the MCP joints of the ring and little fingers.

C True It is also seen in people with epilepsy and cirrhosis of the liver.

D True

E True They lie closely related to the palmar aponeurosis.

12.21 A True The space is divided into compartments by fibrous septa and contains compact fat.

B False The compartment is closed proximally by a fibrous partition from the deep fascia attached to the periosteum distal to the attachment of the flexor tendon.

C True This is due to the presence of unyielding fat and fibrous tissue in the space. Pain is worse at night.

C False The periosteum is left intact.

D False The proximal part, which has an epiphysis and a separate blood supply, is not affected because the space is distal.

12.22 Regarding mallet finger:
    A   Flexor digitorum profundus is ruptured.
    B   It is associated with avulsion fracture of the distal tip of the distal phalanx.
    C   The distal phalanx is kept flexed.
    D   There is inability for passive extension.
    E   It can be treated without suturing the ruptured tendon.

12.23 The neck of the femur:
    A   Is bounded posteriorly by the intertrochanteric line.
    B   Is wholly intracapsular.
    C   Is closely related to the obturator externus muscle.
    D   May lead to avascular necrosis when fractured.
    E   Causes medial rotation of the thigh when fractured.

12.24 The lesser trochanter of the femur:
    A   Receives attachment of the abductors of the hip joint.
    B   Receives attachment of the lateral rotators of the hip.
    C   Has the psoas major attached to it.
    D   Is palpable.
    E   Has a growth plate which is intracapsular.

(Answers overleaf)

12.22 A False The deformity is produced by rupture of the terminal slip of the extensor digitorum, which is often due to forced flexion of the distal phalanx while the extensor is contracting.
  B False The extensor digitorum slip is attached to the dorsal aspect of the proximal end of the distal phalanx. Bone may be fractured at the point of attachment.
  C True It is held in about 30° of flexion.
  D False Active extension is lost; passive extension is possible.
  E True Provided the fractured bone is not markedly displaced, the tendon will heal well if the phalanx is splinted in full extension.

12.23 A False The intertrochanteric line lies anteriorly; and the intertrochanteric crest lies posteriorly.
  B False Posteriorly, the capsule is attached half-way along the neck.
  C True The muscle winds round the inferior aspect of the neck.
  D True The blood supply to the head passes through the retinacula on the neck.
  E False Marked lateral rotation of the thigh is a sign of fractured neck of femur.

12.24 A False The gluteus medius and minimus (abductors) are inserted into the greater trochanter.
  B False The obturators and piriformis are inserted into the greater trochanter; quadratus femoris is inserted into the quadrate tubercle.
  C True The iliacus is also attached.
  D False The greater trochanter is palpable.
  E False The growth plate for the head of the femur is intracapsular while that of the lesser trochanter and most of the growth plate for the greater trochanter are extracapsular.

12.25 Regarding the shaft of the femur:
A   The linea aspera is on its posterior aspect.
B   The vastus intermedius is attached to the linea aspera.
C   It is closely related to the perforating arteries.
D   Displacement is rare when fractured.
E   When fractured, bleeding can occur without visible swelling or bruising.

12.26 Regarding the patella:
A   It is stabilized against displacement by greater prominence of the lateral condyle.
B   It receives attachment of the vastus medialis.
C   It dislocates to the medial side of the knee.
D   Displacement of fragments always follows fracture.
E   Active extension may still be possible after a transverse fracture.

12.27 Regarding the tibia and fibula:
A   The femur articulates with their upper ends.
B   The talus articulates with their lower ends.
C   Fracture of the shaft of the tibia is always associated with significant angulation and displacement.
D   Fracture of the shaft of the tibia is often compound.
E   Delayed union is unlikely if the shaft of the tibia is fractured with the fibula remaining intact.

(Answers overleaf)

12.25 A True This linear ridge receives many muscle attachments.
B False It is attached to the anterior surface of the shaft.
C True These are close to the shaft as they run from the extensor (anterior) compartment to the flexor (posterior) compartment.
D False Displacement occurs because of muscle contraction. When the upper third is fractured, the upper fragment is flexed (iliopsoas) and abducted (gluteus medius and minimus) and the lower fragment is adducted and drawn proximally (producing a shortening). When the middle or lower third is fractured the lower fragment is displaced posteriorly.
E True More than a litre of blood can be lost because of avulsion of arteries close to the bone. This may cause haemorrhagic shock.

12.26 A True Those with an unusually low lateral condyle are more prone to patellar dislocation.
B True The fleshy fibres are attached to the medial border and they prevent lateral displacement.
C False It dislocates laterally by the direction of pull of the quadriceps, which is upwards and lateral.
D False Transverse fracture can occur without displacement, the fragments being held together by the quadriceps tendon and the patellar retinacula.
E True Active extension, though painful, is still possible if the displacement of fragments is minimal.

12.27 A False The lower end of the femur articulates with the tibia to form the knee joint. The upper end of the fibula articulates with the tibia and is outside the knee joint.
B True The lower ends of the tibia and fibula together with the medial and lateral malleoli form the mortise for the ankle joint.
C False Displacement and angulation is minimal if the fibula is not fractured. The intact fibula will act as a strut.
D True It is more commonly compound than fractures of any other bone. This is because the anterior border and the medial surface of the shaft are subcutaneous. This will make skin closure difficult.
E False Delayed union is not uncommon, which may be because the intact fibula is acting as a strut preventing the fragments coming into close contact.

12.28 Regarding rupture of the Achilles tendon:
  A   A gap is felt at the site of rupture.
  B   It usually occurs in elderly men and women.
  C   It is associated with fracture of the os calcis.
  D   Dorsiflexion is limited.
  E   Plantar flexion is completely absent.

12.29 The hip joint owes its stability to:
  A   The diameter of the femoral head being greater than the rim of the acetabular labrum.
  B   A thick and tight fibrous capsule.
  C   The tautness of the iliofemoral ligament in extension.
  D   The strength of the ligament of the head of the femur.
  E   The short lateral rotators of the femur.

12.30 In posterior dislocation of the hip:
  A   It may be associated with fracture of the posterior rim of the acetabulum.
  B   The head of the femur is felt in the gluteal region.
  C   The leg is externally rotated.
  D   A radiograph will show alteration of Shenton's line.
  E   The sciatic nerve should be tested before reduction.

(Answers overleaf)

12.28 A   True   The tendon is subcutaneous.
     B   False   It usually occurs in middle-aged men. It is the commonest tendon to rupture.
     C   False   The tendon ruptures following a trivial stumble, possibly because the tendon is relatively ischaemic and weak.
     D   False   Dorsiflexion is exaggerated because it is normally limited by the tension of the Achilles tendon.
     E   False   Plantar flexion is limited and the patient is unable to stand on tiptoe. However, some plantar flexion is still possible owing to the action of the long flexors of the toes, tibialis posterior and the peronei.

12.29 A   True   The bony surfaces make a good fit, as the smaller size of the rim prevents the head from slipping out of the acetabulum.
     B   True   The capsule is thicker and tighter than that of the shoulder joint.
     C   True   The capsule and the ligaments are taut and the joint is in the stable position when it is extended and medially rotated. The iliofemoral ligament resists the weight of the body which tends to extend the pelvis on the femora in the standing position.
     D   True
     E   True   These muscles are closely related to the capsule and they tend to prevent excessive medial rotation in walking and running.

12.30 A   True   As the hip joint is very stable, only violent trauma will produce dislocation and it may be associated with acetabular fracture and knee injuries.
     B   False   The head of the femur is not palpable because of the overlying soft tissue.
     C   False   The leg is flexed, internally rotated and adducted following a posterior dislocation.
     D   True   Shenton's line is a curved line formed by the superior ramus of the pubis, the head of the femur and the femoral neck.
     E   True   The sciatic nerve lies posterior to the hip joint and may be injured.

12.31 During exposure of the hip joint:
  A   Gluteus medius is encountered in the anterolateral approach.
  B   Gluteus maximus is encountered in the posterior approach.
  C   No significant artery or nerve is encountered in the anterolateral approach.
  D   The sciatic nerve is vulnerable.
  E   The short lateral rotators are cut to expose the posterior aspect of the capsule.

12.32 Regarding the knee joint:
  A   The posterior cruciate ligament is attached to the lateral femoral condyle.
  B   The lateral meniscus is attached to the lateral collateral ligament.
  C   It is supplied by branches from the femoral and sciatic nerves.
  D   The patella moves upwards and laterally during extension.
  E   Medial rotation of the femur occurs when it extends on the tibia.

12.33 The anterior cruciate ligament:
  A   Is attached to the anterior part of the intercondylar area of the tibia.
  B   Is attached to the medial surface of the lateral condyle of the femur.
  C   Is taut in full extension.
  D   Prevents the tibia from sliding excessively forwards on the femur.
  E   Is intrasynovial.

(Answers overleaf)

12.31 A True   The approach is usually through the interval between the gluteus medius and the tensor fasciae latae.

B True   It is split in the direction of its fibres.

C False   The ascending branch of the lateral circumflex artery and the accompanying veins are ligated. The nerve to tensor fasciae latae is also encountered.

D True   The sciatic nerve lies behind the hip joint, separated from the capsule by the short lateral rotators. The nerve is vulnerable when the femoral head is dislocated in order to remove it so that it can be replaced by a prosthesis.

E True   The piriformis, obturator internus and the gemelli which lie on the posterior surface of the capsule are divided.

12.32 A False   The posterior cruciate ligament is attached to the medial femoral condyle, and the anterior cruciate to the lateral femoral condyle.

B False   The lateral meniscus is attached to the popliteus and it is free to move. The medial meniscus is fixed as it is adherent to the deep part of the medial collateral ligament. The medial meniscus is more prone to injury.

C True   It is also supplied by the obturator nerve.

D True   This is by the pull of the quadriceps which is upwards and lateral. When the patella dislocates, it dislocates upwards and laterally.

E True   This 'screw home' movement makes the capsule and the ligaments tight and the knee stable. At the beginning of flexion the femur is rotated laterally by the popliteus to unwind the capsule and the ligaments.

12.33 A True   The cruciate ligaments are named after their tibial attachments.

B True   It crosses in front of the posterior cruciate ligament.

C True   Forced hyperextension can rupture the ligament.

D True   When the ligament is ruptured, the tibia slides excessively forward on the femur when pulled.

E False   Both the cruciate ligaments are extrasynovial.

12.34 Regarding the ankle joint:
  A   Maximal stability is in dorsiflexion.
  B   The deltoid ligament is attached to the sustentaculum tali.
  C   An inversion injury may fracture both the malleoli.
  D   An eversion injury may rupture the deltoid ligament.
  E   It is best aspirated anteriorly.

12.35 Regarding the neuromuscular junction:
  A   Each muscle fibre has many neuromuscular junctions.
  B   Each alpha motor neuron axon innervates many muscle cells.
  C   Acetylcholine is the neurotransmitter at the neuromuscular junction.
  D Ca^{++} ions are involved in release of acetylcholine into the synaptic cleft.
  E   Influx of Na^+ into the muscle depolarizes the muscle fibre.

12.36 Regarding the cellular basis of muscle contraction:
  A   Lining membrane of the muscle fibre is called sarcomere.
  B   On stimulation, extracellular calcium enters the muscle cells to produce contraction.
  C   Sarcoplasmic reticulum contains calcium ions.
  D   T-tubules are connected to the sarcoplasmic reticulum.
  E   Myoglobin converts adenosine diphosphate (ADP) to adenosine triphosphate (ATP).

(Answers overleaf)

12.34 A True This is because the articular surface of the talus is wider anteriorly.

B True It is attached above to the medial malleolus and below to the talus, sustentaculum tali and the spring ligament.

C True The lateral malleolus is fractured because of traction and the medial malleolus by compression force.

D True This is due to traction force and the compression force can fracture the lower end of the fibula.

E True The joint is entered between the tendons of tibialis anterior and extensor hallucis longus.

12.35 A False Each muscle fibre has only one neuromuscular junction.

B True The alpha motor neuron and the muscle fibres it innervates constitute a motor unit.

C True Acetylcholine is synthesized in the cytoplasm of the neuron and is stored as vesicles at the nerve terminal.

D True Arrival of an action potential at the nerve terminal opens up voltage-activated calcium channels. The resulting increase in intracellular calcium will make the acetylcholine vesicles fuse with the presynaptic membrane and release acetylcholine into the synaptic cleft.

E True This produces the end-plate potential. Acetylcholine binds to the nicotinic acetylcholine receptors at the postsynaptic membrane causing the influx of Na^+.

12.36 A False Sarcomeres are repeating units of contractile proteins consisting of thick filaments (myosin) and thin filaments (actin). Sarcolemma is the cell membrane of the muscle cell.

B False Calcium is stored in the sarcoplasmic reticulum and is released into the cytoplasm. Calcium binds to troponin, a protein bound to actin, causing movement of tropomyosin, a protein covering the myosin-binding sites on actin. Myosin heads get attached to these sites causing sliding movement which is magnified into contraction of the muscle fibre.

C True

D True They are also connected to the sarcolemma. Activation of sarcolemma activates the T-tubules and the sarcoplasmic reticulum to release calcium into the cytoplasm.

E False Hydrolysis of ATP to ADP powers muscle contraction. Myoglobin is an oxygen-binding protein. A good blood supply and myoglobin are essential for oxidative phosphorylation of ADP to ATP.

12.37 Regarding skeletal muscle fibre types:
   A   Type I fibres fatigue quickly.
   B   Type IIB fibres are red oxidative type containing more myoglobin.
   C   Type I fibres have high glycogen content.
   D   Muscle fibres within the same motor unit are of the same type.
   E   Type I fibres are innervated by small motor neurons.

12.38 Regarding bone tissue:
   A   The major protein is collagen.
   B   It is synthesized by osteocytes.
   C   Osteocytes are interlinked by their processes.
   D   Osteoclasts resorb bone.
   E   Parathormone promotes the synthesis of bone by osteoblasts.

12.39 Regarding endochondral ossification:
   A   It occurs in all long bones except the clavicle.
   B   The primary centres appear in utero.
   C   Epiphyses are all present at birth.
   D   Epiphyseal cartilage (growth plate) separates the diaphysis from the metaphysis.
   E   Epiphyseal cartilage is involved in increasing length and width of long bones.

(Answers overleaf)

12.37 A **False** Type I fibres contract slowly and fatigue slowly. Their energy is derived by oxidative phosphorylation. and hence they contain more myoglobin. They form the red muscle fibres.

   B **False** They are fast-contracting muscle fibres whose energy source is glycolysis. They have less myoglobin as the contraction is anaerobic.

   C **False** Type IIB has more glycogen, which is their energy source.

   D **True** Fibre types are never mixed within motor units.

   E **True** Slow muscle fibres (type I) are innervated by small motor neurons and faster ones (type IIA and type IIB) by larger neurons.

12.38 A **True** The major protein in the bone matrix is type I collagen. Type I collagen and osteocalcin form the osteoid on which mineralization occurs when the calcium and phosphate levels are normal.

   B **False** The osteoblasts synthesize bone matrix. Osteoblasts get trapped within bone in lacunae and become osteocytes. Osteocytes maintain bone structure.

   C **True** They are interlinked by their processes in canaliculi.

   D **True** They break down bone matrix by lysosomal action and release calcium.

   E **False** Parathormone stimulates bone resorption by osteoclasts.

12.39 A **True** Clavicle is ossified in membrane.

   B **True**

   C **False** Most epiphyses start ossifying after birth from secondary centres.

   D **False** It separates the epiphysis from the metaphysis; metaphysis being the epiphyseal end of the diaphysis.

   E **False** It is involved only in the growth in length; growth in thickness is by subperiosteal deposition of bone.

12.40 Complications of fractures include:
A   Avascular necrosis.
B   Compartment syndrome.
C   Rheumatoid arthritis.
D   Sudeck's atrophy.
E   Deep vein thrombosis.

12.41 During fracture healing:
A   Haematoma is invaded by granulation tissue.
B   Callus is formed around each fragment.
C   Cartilaginous tissue is not formed.
D   Osteoblasts are formed by squamous metaplasia.
E   Callus is not replaced by Haversian bone.

12.42 Regarding osteomyelitis:
A   The usual pathogen is *Staphylococcus aureus*.
B   It begins in the epiphysis.
C   Infarcted bone is called an involucrum.
D   It may infect the growth plate.
E   It may cause pyogenic arthritis.

(Answers overleaf)

12.40 A   True   It occurs in head of femur, proximal half of scaphoid and in the body of talus after fractures of the neck of femur, waist of scaphoid and the neck of the talus respectively.

B   True   It is common in the forearm and leg where there are unyielding compartments, containing muscles, blood vessels and nerves, bounded by bones, interosseus membrane and investing layer of deep fascia.

C   False   Osteoarthritis may complicate intra-articular fractures which cause damage to the articular cartilage; avascular necrosis also can lead on to osteoarthritis.

D   True   This is an occasional late complication and is associated with osteoporosis, soft tissue thickness and vascular stasis along with pain and joint stiffness.

E   True   It is more common in the pelvis and the lower extremity and may be caused by stasis due to compression or immobilization and also due to increased coagulability following operation or injury.

12.41 A   True   Macrophages and other inflammatory cells invade the blood clot and convert it into granulation tissue.

B   True   The osteoprogenitor cells in the periosteum and endosteum are stimulated to form a callus collar around each fragment and they then grow towards each other.

C   False   Osteoprogenitor cells close to the shaft receiving abundant blood supply are converted to osteoblasts which give rise to bony trabeculae anchoring the callus to the shaft. The osteoprogenitor cells further away from the shaft have relatively less blood supply and are converted to chondrocytes. The cartilaginous part of the callus undergoes ossification.

D   False   They are formed by conversion of osteoprogenitor cells.

E   False   The woven bone formed in the callus is remodelled to form Haversian systems to complete the healing process.

12.42 A   True   *Haemophilus influenzae* and streptococci may occur in children. Chronic osteomyelitis, including that around surgical implants, may involve varying pathogens.

B   False   A common site is the metaphysis except in osteomyelitis complicating bone trauma.

C   False   Infarcted bone is called the sequestrum. It stimulates periosteum and new bone formation, and the new bone surrounding the sequestrum is known as involucrum.

D   False   The infection will not invade the growth plate as it is avascular.

E   True   This happens where the metaphysis is intracapsular, as in the hip joint.

12.43   Features of osteoarthritis include:
A   Fibrillation of the articular cartilage.
B   Bone cyst formation.
C   Formation of osteophytes.
D   Fibrosis of the joint capsule.
E   Pannus formation.

12.44   Features of rheumatoid arthritis include:
A   Appearance in childhood.
B   Affecting men more than women.
C   No involvement of the articular cartilage.
D   Narrowing of the joint space.
E   Muscle wasting.

12.45   Metastatic bone tumours:
A   Are rare compared to primary tumours.
B   Chiefly originate from the gastrointestinal tract.
C   Are always of osteolytic type.
D   May present without an obvious primary tumour.
E   May present as a fracture.

12.46   Regarding primary malignant bone tumours:
A   They mostly spread through the lymphatics.
B   Osteosarcoma commonly affects the epiphysis.
C   Chondrosarcoma may have a benign origin.
D   Chondrosarcomas are common in childhood.
E   Ewing's sarcoma occurs in childhood.

(Answers overleaf)

12.43 A **True** Fibrillation is characterized by roughening and fissuring of the articular cartilage. This can lead on to eburnation which exposes the bone surface.
  B **True** Subchondral bone shows sclerosis and cyst formation.
  C **True** They are produced by new bone formation at the periphery of the articular surface.
  D **True** The capsule gets thicker and it undergoes fibrosis causing joint stiffness. Pain in osteoarthritis is caused by capsule and bone involvement. The articular cartilage is not innervated.
  E **False** Pannus is a feature of rheumatoid arthritis.

12.44 A **True** Unlike osteoarthritis, rheumatoid arthritis has a juvenile form known as Still's disease.
  B **False** In Britain it affects about 3% of the female population and 1% of the male population.
  C **False** The disease primarily affects the synovial membrane but progresses to destroy the cartilage; adjacent bone also is eroded.
  D **True** This is similar to osteoarthritis.
  E **True** Pain and movement limitation lead to wasting of muscles and deformities.

12.45 A **False** Metastatic bone tumours (secondary tumours) occur more frequently than primary tumours.
  B **False** They originate far more commonly from the breast, prostate, bronchus and kidney. Follicular carcinoma of the thyroid also metastasizes to bone.
  C **False** The majority are of the osteolytic type, but osteosclerotic (osteoblastic) tumours also occur, such as those from the prostate.
  D **True**
  E **True** Malignancy may be overlooked unless a detailed history is taken and X-rays are examined carefully.

12.46 A **False** Spread is through the bloodstream, mostly to the lungs.
  B **False** They occur in the metaphyses commonly at the lower end of the femur or at the upper end of the tibia.
  C **True** Usually they start in the bone. Hip bone and ribs are commonly affected. Occasionally the tumour may start as a benign lesion.
  D **False** They are more common in the 35–55 age group.
  E **True** They occur more frequently in children and in adolescents. The middle of the shaft of long bones is affected.

12.47   Regarding metabolic diseases of bone:
    A   Osteoporosis is always associated with endocrine abnormality.
    B   Early osteoporotic changes can be detected radiologically.
    C   Osteoporotic fractures are more common in the shaft of long bones.
    D   Osteomalacia is due to deficiency of vitamin A absorption.
    E   Osteomalacia shows Looser's zone on X-ray.

(Answers overleaf)

12.47 A   False   Though thyroid, pituitary and parathyroid diseases cause osteoporosis, it is also associated with gastrointestinal disorders, malignancy, chronic bronchitis and rheumatoid arthritis. It can also be caused by steroid therapy as well as treatment with anticonvulsants and anticoagulants.

B   False   Changes are not obvious until there is about 40% bone loss.

C   False   Cancellous bone is more affected and the fractures are more common in vertebral body, neck of femur and distal radius.

D   False   It is due to a defect in the formation and metabolism of vitamin D_3, which acts with parathyroid hormone to maintain the calcium level.

E   True   They appear as transverse radiolucent lines surrounded by a small amount of sclerotic bone. They can be mistaken for stress fractures.

13. Head and neck

13.1 With regard to the mandible:
A The submandibular gland lies entirely below the mylohyoid line.
B The lingual nerve is closely related to the last molar tooth.
C Fractures of the body are always compound fractures.
D Fractures of the angle are always associated with displacement.
E Fracture of the neck can result in dislocation of the temporomandibular joint.

13.2 The common carotid artery:
A Is contained within the carotid sheath.
B Lies lateral to the internal jugular vein.
C Is closely related to the sympathetic trunk.
D Has no side branches.
E Terminates at the upper border of the thyroid cartilage.

13.3 The internal jugular vein:
A Is a continuation of the sigmoid sinus.
B At its commencement, lies behind the internal carotid artery.
C May be cannulated by inserting the needle between sternal and clavicular heads of the sternocleidomastoid.
D Has the middle thyroid vein as a tributary.
E Is closely associated with lymph nodes.

13.4 The posterior triangle contains:
A The accessory nerve.
B The branches of the cervical plexus.
C The external jugular vein.
D The internal jugular vein.
E Lymph nodes.

(Answers overleaf)

13.1   **A**   **False**   The deep part of the gland lies above the mylohyoid muscle in the oral cavity.
B   **True**   Nerve damage is common during difficult extraction of the tooth.
C   **True**   The mucous membrane is closely adherent to the bone.
D   **False**   If the fracture line is downwards and forwards, the two fragments are impacted and displacement is prevented. If the fracture is downwards and backwards, the posterior fragment is displaced upwards by muscular contraction.
E   **True**   The lateral pterygoid will pull the upper fragment forward dislocating the joint.

13.2   **A**   **True**   The carotid sheath also contains the internal jugular vein and the vagus nerve.
B   **False**   The vein is lateral to the artery with the vagus nerve between the two.
C   **True**   The sympathetic trunk lies closely behind the carotid sheath.
D   **True**
E   **True**   But sometimes the division can be at a higher level, a point worth remembering to avoid inadvertent ligation of the common carotid artery instead of the external carotid.

13.3   **A**   **True**
B   **True**   The vein lies lateral to the carotids as it descends.
C   **True**   It can also be cannulated at a higher level by inserting the needle lateral to the carotid pulsation deep to the anterior border of the sternocleidomastoid at the level of C6 vertebra.
D   **True**   The middle thyroid veins may vary in number. They are short and thin walled and undue traction can avulse them and the internal jugular vein during thyroid surgery.
E   **True**   The deep cervical nodes lie on the vein and may become adherent to it if involved in malignancy or inflammation.

13.4   **A**   **True**   It lies along a line extending from the junction between the upper and middle third of the posterior border of the sternocleidomastoid to a point 5 cm above the lower end of the anterior border of the trapezius.
B   **True**   They emerge at the posterior border of the sternocleidomastoid just below the accessory nerve.
C   **True**   It drains into the subclavian vein at the root of the neck.
D   **False**   This lies deep to the sternocleidomastoid nearer to its anterior border.
E   **True**   The accessory nerve can be damaged during biopsy of a lymph node causing paralysis of the trapezius.

13.5   With regard to the tongue:
  A   The hypoglossal nerve supplies the extrinsic muscles.
  B   Lymphatics from the whole of one side drain into the submandibular lymph nodes.
  C   It has two lingual veins draining it on each side.
  D   A lingual thyroid may occasionally be present at the foramen caecum.
  E   The posterior third has a nerve supply from the glossopharyngeal nerve.

13.6   The parotid gland:
  A   Extends behind the temporomandibular joint.
  B   Has a duct which is palpable.
  C   Is well encapsulated.
  D   Has the retromandibular vein in its substance.
  E   Receives secretomotor fibres from the facial nerve.

13.7   The following are at risk during surgery of the submandibular gland:
  A   The glossopharyngeal nerve.
  B   The facial artery.
  C   The hypoglossal nerve.
  D   The lingual nerve.
  E   The mandibular branch of the facial nerve.

(Answers overleaf)

13.5   **A**   **True**   It supplies the extrinsic and intrinsic muscles except the palatoglossus.

         B   **False**   The posterior third drains into the deep cervical nodes.

         C   **True**   One accompanies the lingual artery in the substance of the tongue and the other lies along the inferior surface.

         D   **True**   The thyroid gland develops from the thyroglossal duct which commences at this point.

         E   **True**   The nerve also supplies the oropharynx.

13.6   **A**   **True**   The superior surface is behind the joint and is closely related to the external auditory meatus.

         B   **True**   It can be palpated on a clenched masseter. It opens opposite the second upper molar tooth in the vestibule.

         C   **True**   Enlargement stretches the capsule, which is innervated by the great auricular nerve, along which the pain sensation may be transmitted causing ear ache.

         D   **True**   Structures within the gland from superficial to deep are the facial nerve, retromandibular vein, and external carotid artery.

         E   **False**   Secretomotor innervation is through fibres in the glossopharyngeal nerve which synapse in the otic ganglion.

13.7   **A**   **False**   The nerve lies deep to the hyoglossus and is not vulnerable.

         B   **True**   The artery is embedded in the posterior aspect of the gland and partly lies deep to the gland.

         C   **True**   The nerve is closely related to the deep part of the gland deep to the mylohyoid.

         D   **True**   The submandibular duct winds round the lingual nerve.

         E   **True**   It lies on the surface of the gland as it loops down below the mandible.

13.8   The palatine tonsil:
A   Is contained inside a fascial capsule.
B   Has its blood supply from the tonsillar branch of the facial artery.
C   Has venous drainage to the paratonsillar vein.
D   Has lymphatic drainage to the jugulodigastric lymph nodes.
E   Has sensory innervation by the vagus nerve.

13.9   The following statements about the piriform fossa are true:
A   It lies within the larynx.
B   It is related to Killian's dehiscence.
C   Malignant tumours may be silent in the early stages.
D   It is supplied by the recurrent laryngeal nerve.
E   The lymphatics drain into the deep cervical nodes.

13.10 Concerning the larynx:
A   The vocal cords are abducted by the cricothyroid muscles.
B   The whole laryngeal mucosa is covered by respiratory epithelium.
C   It has a submucous space throughout.
D   In an emergency, laryngotomy is done by making an opening in the cricothyroid ligament to relieve airway obstruction.
E   Carcinoma of the vocal cords spreads to the regional lymph nodes in the early stage.

(Answers overleaf)

13.8 **A** **False** The capsule separates the deep surface from the underlying superior constrictor muscle. The inner surface is lined by the mucous membrane of the oropharynx with stratified squamous epithelium.

B **True** This is the main blood supply. It also receives branches from the lingual, ascending pharyngeal and ascending palatine arteries.

C **False** Drainage is mostly to the pharyngeal plexus of veins. The paratonsillar vein lying deep to the tonsil may bleed during tonsillectomy.

D **False** The glossopharyngeal nerve is the sensory nerve of the tonsil and the tonsillar fossa. There may be a small contribution from the lesser palatine nerves.

E **True** The node may be palpable behind the angle of the mandible in chronic tonsillitis.

13.9 **A** **False** It is a part of the laryngeal part of the pharynx seen as a cul-de-sac in its anterolateral part.

B **False** Killian's dehiscence is in the midline posteriorly on the pharyngeal wall where the thyropharyngeal fibres diverge from the cricopharyngeus muscle. It is the weakest part of the pharyngeal wall and the site of pharyngeal diverticula.

C **True** They do not cause dysphagia or pressure symptoms.

D **False** It is supplied by the internal laryngeal nerve which lies just under the mucosa before entering the larynx.

E **True** It has a rich lymphatic drainage. Malignant tumours metastasize into the deep cervical nodes in the early stage.

13.10 **A** **False** They are abducted by the posterior cricoarytenoid muscles. The cricothyroid muscles lengthen the cords. All the intrinsic muscles of the larynx are innervated by the recurrent laryngeal nerve except the cricothyroid which is supplied by the external laryngeal nerve.

B **False** The vocal cords have stratified squamous epithelium.

C **False** At the vocal cords the mucosa is firmly adherent to the underlying structures without a submucous space. In laryngeal oedema, fluid accumulates in the submucous space in the supraglottic region causing airway obstruction. Fluid cannot spread downwards because of the absence of submucous space at the cords.

D **True** This opening will be below the level of the vocal cords and can be life-saving.

E **False** As the vocal cords have no lymphatics, the tumour will remain locally malignant for a long while before metastasizing.

13.11 Concerning the nasal cavity and nasopharynx:
- A   The auditory tube opens into the nasopharynx.
- B   The most expanded part is the superior meatus.
- C   The maxillary sinus opens into the middle meatus.
- D   The nasal cavity is supplied entirely by branches of the external carotid artery.
- E   Unilateral deafness without pain in the ear may be due to a tumour in the nasopharynx.

13.12 With regard to the paranasal sinuses:
- A   The frontal and ethmoidal sinuses are closely related to the frontal lobe of the brain.
- B   The maxillary sinus has an opening in its most dependent part.
- C   The maxillary sinus is closely related to the upper molar teeth.
- D   Carcinoma of the maxillary sinus may spread into the orbit.
- E   The sphenoidal sinus is closely related to the pituitary gland.

13.13 Regarding the stellate ganglion:
- A   It is the only ganglion on the cervical part of the sympathetic trunk.
- B   It lies anterior to the neck of the first rib.
- C   It is related anteriorly to the vertebral artery.
- D   It supplies postganglionic fibres to the upper limb.
- E   Blockage or removal of the ganglion produces Horner's syndrome.

(Answers overleaf)

13.11 A **False** The auditory (Eustachian) tube connects the middle ear to the nasopharynx. Its opening is bounded behind by the tubal elevation, which may be used as a landmark in identifying the opening during catheterization of the auditory tube.

   B **False** The most expanded part is the inferior meatus through which nasal intubations are done.

   C **True** It opens into the middle meatus along with the frontal and ethmoidal sinuses. Infection from one sinus can spread to the others because of the proximity of these openings.

   D **False** The anterior and posterior ethmoidal arteries which are branches of the ophthalmic artery also supply the nasal cavity.

   E **True** The tumour blocks the auditory tube.

13.12 A **True** Infection or tumour can spread into the brain.

   B **False** The opening is towards the upper part of its medial wall and is inefficiently placed for drainage.

   C **True** A bad extraction can cause an antro-oral fistula. The teeth and the sinus are supplied by the superior dental nerves and hence infection of one can cause referred pain in the other.

   D **True** The orbit lies above the sinus. Spread to the orbit may cause pain and epiphora and diplopia due to involvement of extraocular muscles.

   E **True** The pituitary gland lies above the sinus and can be surgically approached through the nasal cavity and the sphenoidal sinus.

13.13 A **False** There are three ganglia in the neck – the superior, middle and inferior cervical ganglia. The inferior ganglion is fused with the first thoracic ganglion to form the stellate ganglion.

   B **True** It is also in front of the transverse process of the seventh cervical vertebra.

   C **True** It is related also to the subclavian artery and the apex of the lung and pleura.

   D **True** It also supplies postganglionic fibres to the head and neck. All the preganglionic fibres to the other cervical ganglia pass through the stellate ganglion. Therefore its removal denervates the head and neck of its sympathetic supply.

   E **True** The syndrome is characterized by ptosis, miosis and anhydrosis on the side of the lesion.

13.14 The following statements regarding cervical lymph nodes are true:

A   The superior group of deep cervical nodes lies where the posterior belly of the digastric crosses the internal jugular vein.

B   The lower deep cervical nodes drain the posterior third of the tongue.

C   The submandibular nodes lie within the capsule of the submandibular salivary gland.

D   Infection of the scalp spreads to the parotid nodes.

E   Superficial nodes in the posterior triangle lie along the external jugular vein.

13.15 Regarding the eyeball and the optic pathway:

A   The levator palpebrae has a double innervation.

B   The lacrimal sac lies behind the medial palpebral ligament.

C   The aqueous humour is produced in the anterior chamber.

D   The fovea centralis is the blind spot in the optic disc.

E   All the fibres in the optic nerve decussate in the optic chiasma.

(Answers overleaf)

13.14 A True They drain the tonsil and the tongue, and the efferents go to lower deep cervical nodes or to the jugular lymph trunk. This group is closely related to the accessory nerve.

B True This group lies where omohyoid crosses the internal jugular vein. They drain the tongue, oral cavity, trachea, oesophagus and the thyroid gland.

C True They drain the upper lip, lateral part of the lower lip, cheek, gums and the lateral aspect of the anterior two-thirds of the tongue.

D True The parotid nodes drain the scalp and the ear.

E True These lie superficial to the deep fascia and they drain the areas drained by the external jugular vein. The accessory nerve and the supraclavicular nerves are vulnerable during biopsy of these lymph nodes.

13.15 A True Most of it is striated muscle innervated by the oculomotor nerve. The deep part is smooth muscle innervated by the sympathetics.

B True Tension of the ligament during blinking compresses the sac and drains the lacrimal fluid into the nasolacrimal duct and the nasal cavity.

C False It is produced by the ciliary processes in the posterior chamber and enters the anterior chamber through the pupil to be absorbed in the canal of Schlemm at the iridocorneal angle.

D False The fovea centralis is in the macula lutea and is the site of maximum acuity of vision. The optic disc lies nasal to the macula.

E False The medial fibres decussate and continue into the contralateral optic tract; the lateral fibres continue into the ipsilateral optic tract without decussation in the chiasma. Compression of the middle of the chiasma results in bitemporal hemianopia as it affects decussating fibres from the medial half of each retina.

13.16 Regarding the middle ear:
A   A grommet is inserted into the anterior inferior quadrant of the tympanic membrane.
B   The stapedius is supplied by the facial nerve.
C   During transmission of sound by the ossicles, the handle of the malleus and the long process of the incus move in the same direction.
D   Sound pressure is reduced during transmission through the middle ear.
E   Vibrations transmitted by the stapes produce displacement of the basilar membrane.

13.17 The following statements about sialolithiasis are true:
A   Primary calculi are more commonly seen in the submandibular gland ducts than in the parotid.
B   Secondary calculi may be associated with hypercalcaemia.
C   Swelling is recurrent and is associated with meals in the early stages.
D   Calculi are not radio-opaque.
E   Stones are always within the substance of the gland and are not palpable.

13.18 Regarding tumours of the salivary glands:
A   Mixed parotid tumour is benign.
B   Mixed parotid tumour affects the superficial lobe.
C   Warthin's tumour occurs mostly in the submandibular gland.
D   Warthin's tumour shows cystic spaces.
E   Adenocystocarcinoma mostly affects the parotid gland.

(Answers overleaf)

13.16 A True This is to avoid injury of the chorda tympani nerve, which crosses the tympanic membrane in its upper half.

B True In response to a loud sound, the tensor tympani and the stapedius contract to dampen the vibrations. Facial nerve paralysis causes hyperacusis.

C True Medial movement of the tympanic membrane rocks the head of the malleus and the body of the incus laterally, moving the handle of the malleus and the long process of the incus medially.

D False Sound pressure is accentuated 15 to 20 times because it is transmitted from a larger tympanic membrane to a smaller oval window. The vibrations of the ossicles also accentuate it by about 1.3 times.

E True This will initiate movement of the hair cells and tectorial membrane of the organ of Corti to produce impulses in the auditory nerve.

13.17 A True They may be caused by stasis of salivary secretion and changes in its physicochemical characteristics.

B True They are also associated with hyperuricaemia.

C True

D False Calculi are usually radio-opaque.

E False Stones can be anywhere along Wharton's duct or Stensen's duct and may be palpable.

13.18 A True About 70% of the benign salivary gland tumours are of this type.

B True It is well encapsulated and does not involve the facial nerve. Its removal can be done while preserving the facial nerve and its branches.

C False It is rare in the submandibular gland. About 10% of the benign parotid tumours are of this type.

D True It is an adenolymphoma characterized by cystic spaces and lymphoid tissue in between cysts.

E False It affects the submandibular gland more than the parotid. Total eradication by surgical excision is difficult because of extensive infiltration into local tissues.

14. Endocrine system

14.1 Regarding development of the thyroid gland:
A   It is not fully developed at birth.
B   The foramen caecum is a remnant of the thyroglossal duct.
C   A thyroglossal cyst is an embryological remnant.
D   The thyroglossal duct is closely related to the hyoid bone.
E   Patients with lingual thyroid often show signs of hyperthyroidism.

14.2 Regarding the blood supply of the thyroid gland:
A   The external laryngeal nerve is related to the superior thyroid artery pedicle.
B   The inferior thyroid artery is best ligated close to the capsule of the gland.
C   Bilateral ligature of the inferior thyroid artery is recommended in subtotal thyroidectomy.
D   There are more than two inferior thyroid veins.
E   The internal jugular vein can be damaged during ligation of the middle thyroid vein.

14.3 The recurrent laryngeal nerves:
A   Lie in the groove between the trachea and oesophagus.
B   Are related to the anterior surface of the thyroid gland.
C   Are most vulnerable where they cross the inferior constrictor.
D   Have a constant relation to the inferior thyroid artery.
E   If paralysed, cause abduction of the vocal cords.

(Answers overleaf)

14.1 **A** **False** Development starts at 4 weeks of intrauterine life and is complete by 6 weeks.

  B **True** The thyroglossal duct, from the caudal end of which the thyroid is developed, extends from the foramen caecum in the tongue to the neck.

  C **True** It is developed from epithelial remnants in the thyroglossal duct.

  D **True** The cyst, which usually appears in the first decade of life, is in the midline and is attached to the hyoid bone. Removal of the cyst necessitates removal of the body of the hyoid.

  E **False** This may be the only thyroid tissue and the patient is often hypothyroid.

14.2 **A** **True** This supplies the cricothyroid muscle; damage to the nerve can cause change in voice.

  B **True** This is to avoid damage to the recurrent laryngeal nerve and also to minimize ischaemia of parathyroid glands.

  C **False** This will cause ischaemia of the parathyroids.

  D **True** There are many veins and they drain into the subclavian or brachiocephalic vein.

  E **True** This is because the vein is very short. Even traction on the thyroid can tear the internal jugular vein. The middle thyroid vein may be found on only one side or it may be absent, in which case veins from the middle of the gland drain into the superior or inferior thyroid veins.

14.3 **A** **True** However, very occasionally, the right nerve may be non-recurrent and can come straight towards the lower pole of the thyroid from the vagus without lying in the groove between the trachea and the oesophagus.

  B **False** The nerves cross the lower poles of the gland and go posteriorly.

  C **True** Here each nerve is deep to a condensation of fibrous tissue connecting the thyroid gland to the trachea – the ligament of Berry.

  D **False** The relationship is very variable. The nerve may lie closely related to the trunk of the artery or it may pass in between the branches of the artery.

  E **False** The vocal cords will be paralysed. They lie motionless midway between abduction and adduction. A tracheostomy may be needed.

14.4   Regarding the follicular cells of the thyroid gland:
A   They surround colloid.
B   They secrete triiodothyronine (T_3) and tetraiodothyronine (T_4) into the follicle.
C   They secrete thyroglobulin into the bloodstream.
D   Iodine transport across the cell is influenced by thyroid-stimulating hormone (TSH).
E   They produce thyroglobulin.

14.5   Regarding thyroid hormones (T_3 and T_4):
A   They mostly circulate in the free state.
B T_3 is more active than T_4.
C   As a replacement therapy after total thyroidectomy, T_3 is given once a day and T_4 three times a day.
D   Increased levels of T_3/T_4 inhibit the TRH/TSH axis.
E   Long-acting thyroid stimulators (LATS) inhibit TSH.

14.6   Thyroid hormones facilitate:
A   Heat production.
B   Insulin breakdown.
C   Lipolysis.
D   Activity of β-adrenergic receptors.
E   Osteoclastic activity.

(Answers overleaf)

14.4 **A** **True** The cells are cuboidal when the follicle is filled with colloid and the cells are resting, and columnar when they become active.

B **False** T_3 and T_4 are secreted into the bloodstream.

C **False** Thyroglobulin is secreted into the lumen of the follicle.

D **True** This is done against a concentration gradient by an active pump. Iodine concentration in follicular cells is 25–50 times more than that in blood.

E **True** In the cell, iodide is oxidized to iodine and the new iodine formed binds with thyroglobulin (to its tyrosine component) which is also produced within the follicular cell.

14.5 **A** **False** They are mostly bound to thyroxine-binding globulin and albumin. Less than 1% circulates in the free state.

B **True** Intracellular T_3 is obtained by deiodination of T_4.

C **False** The half-life of T_4 is longer (1 week) than that of T_3 (1 day). T_4 can be given as replacement therapy once a day and T_3 three time a day.

D **True** There is negative feedback on the hypothalamus and the pituitary.

E **True** LATS are stimulatory thyroid receptor antibodies which increase the production of hormones, which in turn inhibits TSH.

14.6 **A** **True** They do this by increasing O_2 uptake by the mitochondria and increasing ATP production. Patients with thyrotoxicosis suffer heat intolerance and those who are hypothyroid cannot withstand cold.

B **True** They facilitate glucose absorption from the gut and carbohydrate metabolism. Thyrotoxicosis will unmask diabetes mellitus.

C **True** Fatty acid oxidation is increased. In thyrotoxicosis the cholesterol level is lowered, whereas in myxoedema it is raised.

D **True** This increases the cardiac rate and output. Propranolol (β-adrenergic blocker) is used to control tachycardia in thyrotoxicosis.

E **True** Hypercalcaemia and hypercalciuria are seen in thyrotoxicosis.

14.7   Regarding Graves' disease:
A   It is the commonest cause of thyrotoxicosis.
B   Thyroid-stimulating hormone (TSH) level is elevated.
C   The thyroid gland is of normal size.
D   All cases show ophthalmopathy.
E   It is associated with pretibial myxoedema.

14.8   Regarding treatment of thyrotoxicosis:
A   Surgery is contraindicated when the gland is markedly enlarged.
B ^{131}I is indicated in pregnancy.
C   Thiomides are contraindicated before surgery.
D   Subtotal thyroidectomy eliminates the risk of recurrence.
E   Ophthalmopathy is improved after total thyroidectomy.

14.9   Regarding papillary carcinoma of the thyroid:
A   The incidence is less than that of follicular carcinoma.
B   Peak incidence is in the sixth decade.
C   Early spread to regional lymph nodes can occur.
D   Haematogenous spread is common.
E   Prognosis after treatment is good.

(Answers overleaf)

14.7   **A**   **True**   Some of the other causes are overdose of thyroxine, multinodular goitre, hyperfunctioning adenoma and functioning thyroid carcinoma.

       B   **False**   TSH level may be low. Graves' disease is caused by TSH-receptor site antibody which binds to the thyroid follicular cells and mimics the action of TSH.

       C   **False**   There is diffuse enlargement of the gland.

       D   **False**   Mild cases of ophthalmopathy show lid lag and lid retraction and severe cases are associated with proptosis, keratitis and even blindness.

       E   **True**   This is seen in some cases, not in all.

14.8   **A**   **False**   This is an indication for surgery, the others being ophthalmopathy, pregnancy and cancer.

       B   **False**   Patients are advised against pregnancy within 2 years of ^{131}I treatment.

       C   **False**   The euthyroid state should be achieved before surgery and this is done by blocking with thiomides and if necessary replacement with thyroxine (block and replace). Propranolol is used to control catecholamine effects.

       D   **False**   Recurrence is possible after subtotal thyroidectomy. Increased levels of TSH-receptor antibody will cause hyperactivity of the remaining thyroid tissue.

       E   **True**   There is an immediate improvement of eye signs. Total thyroidectomy also eliminates the risk of recurrence of thyrotoxicosis.

14.9   **A**   **False**   It is the commonest among thyroid cancers.

       B   **False**   Peak incidence is in the third decade; however, the tumour can occur in children and the elderly.

       C   **True**   Pretracheal and paratracheal nodes are affected.

       D   **False**   Follicular tumours can spread through the bloodstream to lungs and bones.

       E   **True**   Prognosis is good. Total thyroidectomy followed by ^{131}I and thyroxine is the standard treatment for well-differentiated thyroid cancer.

14.10 Parathyroid hormone (PTH):
A   Has a half-life of 2–3 days.
B   Stimulates osteoclastic activity.
C   Enhances calcium absorption from the gut.
D   Increases urinary excretion of phosphate.
E   Inhibits bicarbonate resorption in the renal tubules.

14.11 Regarding primary hyperparathyroidism:
A   Blood calcium level is decreased.
B   Renal calculi are common.
C   Bone changes are mostly in the lower extremity.
D   The most common cause is a benign adenoma of the parathyroid gland.
E   Surgery is the treatment of choice.

14.12 Hypoparathyroidism:
A   Can be caused by ligation of the inferior thyroid arteries.
B   Occurs in the diGeorge syndrome.
C   Causes hyperphosphataemia.
D   May show carpopedal spasm.
E   Can be treated by calcium supplement in the diet.

(Answers overleaf)

14.10 **A**   **False**   It has a half-life of only 2–3 minutes. Intracellular stores of PTH are also very limited. When glands are removed or become ischaemic during thyroid surgery, the effects of PTH deficiency are sudden.

     B   **True**   Bone resorption is brought about by acid secretion and by the action of proteases. Serum calcium level is increased.

     C   **False**   This is done by 1,25-dihydroxy-vitamin D which is produced in the renal proximal tubules by the action of PTH.

     D   **True**   PTH acts on the proximal renal tubule. By lowering the phosphate level, Ca^{++} level in blood is increased. PTH also acts on the distal tubules to facilitate resorption of Ca^{++}.

     E   **True**   This results in acidosis which will increase calcium ionization.

14.11 **A**   **False**   It causes hypercalcaemia which is associated with raised PTH levels.

     B   **True**   Patients usually present with complaints associated with renal calculi.

     C   **False**   It is generalized; 'ground-glass' appearance of the skull, loss of lamina dura around the teeth, presence of bone cysts are the usual changes seen.

     D   **True**

     E   **True**   Surgery is to remove the adenoma.

14.12 **A**   **True**   The inferior thyroid arteries supply the parathyroid glands, and bilateral ligation of these during thyroid surgery causes ischaemic changes and hypofunction of the parathyroids.

     B   **True**   In this there is congenital absence of parathyroid glands.

     C   **True**   It also causes hypocalcaemia.

     D   **True**   This is due to reduced calcium levels in the blood. There will also be paraesthesia and it may lead on to convulsions and tetany.

     E   **False**   Immediate treatment is by intravenous infusion of calcium; long-term management includes 1-alpha-dihydroxy-vitamin D and dietary calcium supplement.

14.13 Regarding calcium homeostasis:
  A   The main body store of calcium is bone tissue.
  B   The active form of calcium is bound to albumin.
  C   Calcium levels are regulated by parathyroid hormone, 1,25-dihydroxy-vitamin D and calcitonin.
  D   A deficiency of vitamin D causes osteomalacia.
  E   Calcitonin plays a major role in calcium homeostasis in humans.

14.14 Regarding the adrenal glands:
  A   The right adrenal vein drains into the right renal vein.
  B   They have a portal system of cortical vessels which also supply the medulla.
  C   The medulla is of neural crest origin.
  D   The zona glomerulosa produces aldosterone.
  E   The zona fasciculata and zona reticularis respond to adrenocorticotrophic hormone (ACTH).

(Answers overleaf)

14.13 A True   There are lesser amounts in soft tissues and very little in the intracellular compartment.

B False   The free form of ionized calcium, Ca^{++}, is the active form. Calcium bound to albumin, phosphate and citrate is inactive.

C True   Liver and kidney are involved in the synthesis of 1,25-dihydroxy-vitamin D. Thyrocalcitonin is synthesized by the parafollicular cells (C cells) of the thyroid gland.

D True   At normal levels, vitamin D stimulates osteoblastic activity. However, when the levels are raised it promotes osteoclastic activity resulting in bone resorption and hypercalcaemia. Deficiency of vitamin D causes osteomalacia.

E False   There is no evidence for that in humans. Patients who have had thyroidectomy do not show any evidence of calcitonin defect. Patients with high levels of calcitonin as in medullary carcinoma of the thyroid do not have problems with calcium homeostasis.

14.14 A False   The right adrenal vein is very short and it is difficult to handle surgically as it drains into the inferior vena cava which is in contact with the anterior surface of the gland.

B True   Through this, cortical hormones circulate in the medulla before leaving the gland.

C True   The cortex is of mesodermal origin. Sympathetic preganglionic fibres supply the medulla and come in direct contact with the phaeochromocytes.

D True   This is a thin layer just inside the capsule. Deep to this is the thicker zona fasciculata producing cortisol and deeper still is the reticularis (adjoining the medulla) which produces androgens and cortisol.

E True   Hormones are not stored; they are produced on demand. The zona glomerulosa and aldosterone production are controlled by the renin–angiotensin mechanism.

14.15 Regarding the glucocorticoids:
A   Biologically active forms are bound to albumin or globulin.
B   They are not absorbed through skin on topical application.
C   They can cause bone resorption.
D   Long-term treatment may produce atrophy of the zona fasciculata and zona reticularis of the adrenal cortex.
E   Plasma levels can be determined by a single estimation.

14.16 Regarding the renin–angiotensin mechanism:
A   Renin is produced by the juxtaglomerular apparatus of the kidney.
B   Angiotensin-converting enzyme (ACE) cleaves angiotensinogen to produce angiotensin I.
C   Angiotensin II stimulates aldosterone secretion.
D   ACE inhibitors are ideal for controlling hypertension caused by renal artery stenosis.
E   ACE inhibitors are suited to controlling hypertension in diabetic patients.

(Answers overleaf)

14.15 A False 90% of circulating cortisol (hydrocortisone) is bound to albumin or globulin. This is the biologically inactive form, whereas free cortisol which enters cells to interact with the DNA and affects RNA is the active form.

B False Cortisol is absorbed easily when topically applied as cream on skin.

C True Patients on long-term steroid treatment are prone to vertebral body collapse, fractures and avascular necrosis. Bone matrix is reduced and bone resorption is increased. Steroid excess also potentiates the action of parathormone, facilitating bone resorption. Calcium absorption from the gut is reduced.

D True This is by inhibiting the production of CRH (corticotrophin-releasing hormone) by the hypothalamus and ACTH.

E False Maximum output is in the morning just prior to wakening. Estimations should be done first on wakening and another one later in the day towards the evening.

14.16 A True Its production is stimulated by hyponatraemia, reduction of renal perfusion pressure in the afferent arterioles, and increased catecholamine concentration due to sympathetic stimulation.

B False Renin cleaves angiotensinogen (produced in the liver). ACE, produced mostly in lungs, converts angiotensin I to angiotensin II.

C True Angiotensin II is a powerful vasoconstrictor. It also increases sodium reabsorption in the renal tubules and reduces glomerular filtration.

D False ACE causes a fall in the intraglomerular pressure by reducing efferent arteriolar constriction. This associated with renal artery stenosis may cause acute renal failure.

E True This is because of their efficient vasodilatation effect on the efferent arterioles from the glomerulus.

14.17 Regarding adrenal cortex insufficiency:
   A   It results in hyponatraemia.
   B   The most common cause is Addison's disease.
   C   In primary insufficiency, levels of adrenocorticotrophic hormone (ACTH) are suppressed.
   D   A common cause of secondary insufficiency is glucocorticoid therapy.
   E   Patients on long-term steroid therapy can have an acute adrenal crisis during routine operations.

14.18 Regarding Cushing's syndrome:
   A   It may be caused by adrenal hyperplasia.
   B   It may show raised blood sugar.
   C   It may show reduction in bone density.
   D   If cortisol levels remain high after a dexamethasone suppression test, the fault is in the pituitary–adrenal axis.
   E   If metyrapone raises levels of adrenocorticotrophic hormone (ACTH) the pituitary–adrenal axis is normal.

(Answers overleaf)

14.17 A **True** In the acute state, aldosterone deficiency causes increased excretion of sodium and water causing hyponatraemia, hypovolaemia and hypotension.

B **False** Addison's disease causing primary adrenal insufficiency is rare. Other causes of primary insufficiency are metastatic involvement of the adrenals, autoimmune disease and haemorrhage into the adrenals.

C **False** Primary insufficiency is due to a fault in the adrenals. ACTH levels are raised to counteract this.

D **True** Increased glucocorticoid levels suppress ACTH production and cause hypofunction of the cortex.

E **True** The increased demand for corticoids cannot be met because ACTH levels and corticoid production remain suppressed in these patients. They need additional steroid therapy during the operation and also careful evaluation of their state of hydration, electrolytes and blood pressure preoperatively and postoperatively.

14.18 A **True** It may also be caused by a functioning adenoma, in which case the remaining adrenal tissue will be suppressed. The patient will require steroid treatment following removal of the adenoma.

B **True** Raised cortisol level, which is characteristic of Cushing's syndrome, will facilitate the actions of glucagon and catecholamines. Gluconeogenesis is increased and glucose uptake by muscle and fat is reduced.

C **True** This is due to increased bone resorption and increased activity of parathyroid hormone.

D **True** Normally, administration of steroids should reduce the level of ACTH and the endogenous production of cortisol.

E **True** Metyrapone inhibits cortisol production and causes elevation of ACTH.

14.19 Regarding phaeochromocytoma:
- **A** It is a rare tumour of the adrenal medulla.
- **B** It can be associated with multiple endocrine neoplasia (MEN).
- **C** It may be associated with hypoglycaemia.
- **D** Surgery is the treatment of choice.
- **E** α and β catecholamine levels should be controlled before surgery.

14.20 Regarding insulin:
- **A** Rising blood sugar is associated with a rise in circulating insulin.
- **B** The number of insulin receptors on cells is increased as the insulin level is raised.
- **C** It facilitates glycogen and triglyceride synthesis.
- **D** Patients with end-stage diabetic nephropathy require less insulin than diabetics with normal kidneys.
- **E** Low levels of K^+ stimulate insulin secretion.

(Answers overleaf)

14.19 A True It can also arise in any chromaffin tissue of the sympathetic nervous system.

B True It is associated with a genetic abnormality and may show tumours in the thyroid gland, parathyroid and the mucosa of the oral cavity.

C False Hyperglycaemia is a feature because of raised catecholamine levels.

D True Removal of the tumour will cure the patient. Morbidity and mortality due to surgery are high if the patient is not well prepared preoperatively. Anaesthesia and handling the tumour during surgery can cause adverse cardiovascular responses. During surgery, the tumour is handled as little as possible and the adrenal vein is ligated at the beginning of the procedure to prevent a surge of catecholamines into the bloodstream.

E True Phenoxybenzamine (α blocker) and propranolol are used to fully block the α and β adrenergic effects.

14.20 A True Amino acids, some fatty acids, vagal and β-adrenergic stimulation as well as gut hormones such as secretin also stimulate the secretion of insulin.

B False The number decreases to reduce insulin–receptor interaction and uptake of glucose. Insulin receptors are on many cells including the membranes of fat cells, liver cells and muscle cells.

C True In glycogen synthesis, glucose is converted to glycogen and stored as an energy source. Triglyceride synthesis is facilitated by glucose intake by fat cells. Insulin stimulates lipoprotein lipase activity in breaking down circulating chylomicrons. The fat cells take up the fatty acids and glycerol produced and reconvert them to triglycerides. Insulin inhibits breakdown of triglycerides in adipocytes by inhibiting the action of lipolytic lipase.

D True Insulin is normally broken down in the kidneys. The breakdown is reduced in diabetic nephropathy.

E False Drug therapy lowering K^+ levels inhibits insulin secretion. Insulin lowers extracellular K^+ levels by stimulating the intracellular shift of K^+. Insulin and glucose infusion lowers the K^+ levels in hyperkalaemia due to acute renal failure, septicaemia and shock.

14.21 Hypoglycaemia:
  A   May be caused by strenuous exercise.
  B   May be associated with 'dumping' syndrome.
  C   Causes reduced secretion of insulin.
  D   Stimulates the β-adrenergic mechanism and glucagon production.
  E   Causes reduced production of cortisol.

14.22 Regarding diabetes mellitus:
  A   Cellular uptake of sugar is increased.
  B   Type I diabetes is commoner than type II.
  C   Type I can be managed by dietary controls alone.
  D   The risks of ketoacidosis and hypokalaemia are higher in surgical patients with diabetes.
  E   Long-acting insulin will have peak activity commencing about 2 hours after injection.

(Answers overleaf)

14.21 A   True   Long-distance running can deplete glycogen reserves, causing hypoglycaemia. Insulin secretion falls with lowered blood sugar. However, in insulin-dependent diabetics, continued absorption of injected insulin will lead to sudden hypoglycaemia during such exercise.

B   True   Gastric surgery with drainage may cause rapid overloading of the small intestine with carbohydrates. These, when absorbed, cause excess of insulin secretion causing hypoglycaemia.

C   True   Low blood sugar level switches off insulin secretion.

D   True   Catecholamine stimulates glycolysis (raising glucose levels) as well as glucagon secretion. Hypoglycaemia also has direct action on pancreatic A cells (to secrete glucagon).

E   False   Hypoglycaemia and the adrenergic stimulation increase the ACTH production increasing cortisol levels. This will stimulate gluconeogenesis.

14.22 A   False   Cellular uptake of sugars is markedly diminished because insulin is required for this process. However, tissues contain high amounts of sugars because of the high blood sugar levels and this makes them more vulnerable to infections.

B   False   Type II diabetes affecting an older age group is more common than type I diabetes.

C   False   Type I diabetes is insulin dependent.

D   True   Surgery evokes a glucocorticoid and catecholamine response, stimulating lipolysis and ketone body production. Associated K^+ loss may cause hypokalaemia. Frequent perioperative blood sugar monitoring is essential.

E   False   Most short-acting insulin has peak activity starting about 2 hours after injection and lasting for about 2 hours. The action of long-acting insulin starts 6–8 hours after injection and lasts for up to 12–16 hours.

15. Breast

15.1 Regarding the anatomy and structure of the breast:
A   Ligaments of Astley Cooper connect the pectoral fascia to the skin.
B   The thickness of the glandular tissue is uniform throughout.
C   Lobulation of the glandular tissue is prominent during lactation.
D   Most lymph drains into the axillary nodes.
E   Level II clearance of axillary nodes gives better prognosis than level I clearance.

15.2 Normal structural changes in breast include:
A   Breast tissue regresses soon after birth.
B   Ducts proliferate during each menstrual cycle.
C   Alveolar units regress after menstruation.
D   Ductal sprouting is enhanced during the second trimester.
E   The size increase is maximum in the third trimester.

15.1 **A** **True** Breast has an extensive suspensory mechanism which suspends the breast between skin and the underlying pectoral fascia.

B **False** The thickness of the glandular tissue varies in different parts; in the superolateral quadrant it is greater than elsewhere and extends into the axilla as the 'axillary tail'.

C **True** Indentations develop between lobules making the lobules feel like lumps. During pregnancy, the glandular elements hypertrophy with increase in blood supply making the breast feel full, heavy, tense and often painful.

D **True** The majority of the lymph from the breast enters a node near the first rib, from where it descends to axillary nodes at the levels of the third and fourth ribs and then ascends towards nodes near the second rib. Efferents then form a plexus around the axillary vein and reach the nodes overlying the first rib. Lymph trunks formed from these apical nodes take the lymph to the confluence of the subclavian and jugular veins.

E **True** Axillary clearance of all the lymph nodes is difficult and hazardous. Level I removes the nodes around the axillary vein superficial to the pectoralis minor and also the axillary tail, if present. Level II includes nodes deep to pectoralis minor, and level III nodes up to the apex of the axilla. With level I clearance there is 25% chance of involvement of higher nodes, which falls to about 3% with level II dissection.

15.2 **A** **True** Breast development by epithelial proliferation is facilitated by maternal sex steroids until the seventh month, after which the duct system is arranged into lobules. Proliferation of vesicles, which are precursors of the acini, is under control of the maternal progesterone. After birth, regression occurs because of lack of sex steroids.

B **True** This is influenced by oestrogen and occurs in the proliferative stage of the cycle.

C **True** Alveolar units are influenced by the progesterone from the corpus luteum.

D **False** In the second trimester progesterone levels increase markedly and this will inhibit ductal proliferation, which occurs in the first trimester. Progesterone also increases the growth of supporting tissue and the blood supply.

E **True** The size of the alveoli increases and colostrum is produced during the third trimester.

15.3 Regarding lactation:
A Milk production is controlled by prolactin.
B Prolactin receptors on alveoli are inhibited by oestrogen.
C Colostrum has a high content of fat and carbohydrate.
D Milk let-down from alveoli to the ducts is stimulated by prolactin.
E Suckling stimulates prolactin secretion.

15.4 Precancerous changes in the breast are:
A Fibroadenoma.
B Apocrine metaplasia.
C Sclerosing adenoma.
D Atypical ductal hyperplasia.
E Florid epithelial hyperplasia without atypia.

15.5 Regarding carcinoma in situ (CIS):
A Lobular carcinoma in situ (LCIS) presents as a palpable lump.
B LCIS is rarely bilateral.
C The risk of LCIS developing into invasive cancer is minimal.
D Ductal CIS (DCIS) may show mammographically detectable lesions.
E All DCIS show greater chance of recurrence after conservative surgery.

(Answers overleaf)

15.3 **A** **True** This is produced by the anterior pituitary and is similar in structure to growth hormone.

  B **True** Towards the end of pregnancy when the oestrogen levels are down, the number of prolactin receptors increases.

  C **False** Colostrum contains more protein, lactalbumin, than milk. It also has IgG which is absorbed into the gastrointestinal tract of the newborn.

  D **False** Milk let-down is stimulated by oxytocin, which is released from the posterior pituitary. Oxytocin stimulates the myoepithelial cells of the alveoli and ducts. Suckling is a stimulant for the release of oxytocin.

  E **True** When suckling stops, milk accumulates in the alveoli, which in turn inhibits the production of prolactin.

15.4 **A** **False** Fibroadenomas are benign lesions. They are common and are often solitary. They are influenced by hormones and grow fast during pregnancy, mimicking carcinoma.

  B **False** This also is a benign lesion and is not precancerous.

  C **False** This is caused by proliferation of acini and connective tissue. It shows mitotic activity as well as microcalcification. Clinically and pathologically, the lesion may mimic carcinoma.

  D **True** There is an increased risk (five times) of developing cancer in atypical ductal hyperplasia.

  E **True** The chance of developing malignancy is double that of the general population.

15.5 **A** **False** It is silent, without palpable masses and mammographically detectable lesions.

  B **False** LCIS tends to be bilateral and multifocal.

  C **False** 25% of cases subsequently develop invasive cancer in premenopausal women. LCIS regresses after the menopause.

  D **True** DCIS shows areas of calcification which have characteristic features in mammography.

  E **False** Only the comedo type shows a high incidence of recurrence after conservative surgery.

15.6   Regarding breast carcinoma:
A   It affects 1 in 1000 women in the western world.
B   Long exposure to sex hormones may be an aetiological factor.
C   Stromal reaction contributes to most of the clinical findings.
D   Screening programmes are very effective in detecting the tumour at an early stage.
E   It can recur or metastasize after many years of apparent cure.

15.7   Regarding invasive mammary carcinoma:
A   Ductal carcinomas have better prognosis than tubular carcinomas.
B   Lobular carcinomas have a tendency to affect both breasts.
C   Invasive cribriform carcinoma is histologically similar to tubular carcinoma.
D   Medullary carcinoma tends to occur in the older age group.
E   Ductal carcinoma is confined to the duct cells.

15.8   Regarding the classification and prognostic indicators of breast carcinoma:
A   In the TNM classification T_3 denotes tumour fixed to skin and N_3 means fixed ipsilateral nodes.
B   Involvement of supraclavicular nodes denotes distant metastasis.
C   Presence of oestrogen receptors denotes better prognosis.
D   Mitotic count and pleomorphism are prognostic indicators.
E   Lymphatic invasion and blood vessel invasion at the tumour edge indicate potential for spread.

(Answers overleaf)

15.6 A False The incidence is much higher – 1 in 10.
    B True There is a higher incidence in those who have menarche earlier or menopause late and those who are on hormone replacement treatment for many years.
    C True The palpable lump is due to a fibrous tissue proliferation; peau d'orange is due to dermal oedema; and nipple retraction and skin dimpling are due to shortening of the ligament of Cooper.
    D False Aggressive tumour cells spread very early, before the primary is detected; spread may occur as soon as a few malignant cells (16–32) have developed at the primary site.
    E True Malignant cells may remain dormant for many years and the tumour can recur after 30–40 years of apparent cure.

15.7 A False Ductal carcinomas are more invasive than any other form. Tubular carcinomas have no distant metastatic potential and have better prognosis.
    B True However, prognosis is better than in the ductal type unless both sides are affected simultaneously. Distant metastasis via lymph and bloodstream occurs to the mediastinum, brain and bowel walls.
    C True It has an excellent prognosis even if one or two low axillary lymph nodes are involved.
    D False Medullary carcinoma occurs in younger women and has better prognosis than ductal carcinoma.
    E False The tumour cells do not produce an acinar pattern and are hence called ductal. About three-quarters of invasive carcinomas are of this type and they are also known as 'no special type' because they have a wide range of histological appearances and do not match any of the special types.

15.8 A False T_3 denotes tumour size more than 5 cm and T_4 denotes fixity to skin. N_2 is fixed ipsilateral nodes and N_3 means involvement of internal mammary nodes.
    B True
    C True They are seen in well-differentiated tumours.
    D True
    E True

16. Paediatric disorders

16.1 **During prenatal development:**
A   The notochord gives rise to the vertebral column.
B   Most internal and external structures are developed during the fourth to eighth weeks.
C   The cartilage of the first branchial arch develops into the malleus and incus.
D   The artery of the fourth arch on the left side develops into the arch of the aorta.
E   The ductus arteriosus is developed from the sixth arch artery on the left side.

16.2 **Regarding developmental anomalies:**
A   A sacrococcygeal teratoma is linked with a persistent primitive streak.
B   A low preauricular sinus is superficial and has no internal connection.
C   A branchial fistula is usually seen in the midline in the neck.
D   A branchial fistula opens in the foramen caecum in the tongue.
E   A branchial cyst is a remnant of the third arch.

16.3 **Regarding lingual thyroid and thyroglossal cysts:**
A   Lingual thyroid is seen at the foramen caecum of the tongue.
B   Lingual thyroid maintains normal thyroid functions and hence should not be removed.
C   A thyroglossal cyst can present at any age.
D   A thyroglossal cyst is a midline swelling which moves up when the tongue is protruded.
E   A thyroglossal cyst need not be excised unless it is infected.

(Answers overleaf)

16.1 **A** **False** The vertebrae are developed from the somites formed adjacent to the notochord.

B **True** Any disturbance during this period can cause anomalies of various systems.

C **True** The third middle ear bone, the stapes, is developed from the second arch cartilage. The sixth arch cartilage gives rise to the laryngeal cartilages.

D **True** On the right side, the fourth arch artery forms the right subclavian artery.

E **True** This is why the recurrent laryngeal nerve winds round it. On the right side the nerve is shifted upwards on to the subclavian artery (fourth arch) as the sixth and fifth arch arteries disappear.

16.2 **A** **True** It is a benign tumour in the neonate which may turn malignant and hence should be removed at birth.

B **False** It may have deep internal connection to the first arch and may extend into the middle ear, very close to the facial nerve.

C **False** It is seen at the anterior border of the sternomastoid muscle in its lower part.

D **False** The internal opening is in the tonsillar fossa.

E **False** It is a remnant of the second arch.

16.3 **A** **True** This is the site of development of the thyroglossal duct. The foramen caecum is in the midline at the junction between the anterior two-thirds and the posterior third of the tongue.

B **False** A lingual thyroid is usually hypoplastic and should be removed because it may be affected by various pathology including bleeding and infection.

C **True**

D **True** It usually has connection to the tongue through remnants of the thyroglossal duct.

E **False** It should be excised along with the thyroglossal tract and the mid-portion of the hyoid bone. Excision is more difficult once the cyst is infected.

16.4   Cystic hygroma:
A   Is due to persistent fourth branchial arch derivatives.
B   Is also known as a dermoid cyst.
C   Can be large enough to produce respiratory distress in neonates.
D   May extend into the axilla.
E   Is very likely to resolve spontaneously and therefore excision is not indicated.

16.5   Regarding development of the diaphragm and congenital diaphragmatic hernia:
A   The septum transversum contributes to the peripheral muscular part.
B   The mesentery of the foregut contributes to the anterior part.
C   High mortality rate among neonates with congenital diaphragmatic hernia is due to associated lung hypoplasia.
D   The most common defect is the posterolateral Bochdalek hernia.
E   Morgagni's hernias are small defects close to the sternum.

16.6   Oesophageal atresia may be associated with:
A   Tracheo-oesophageal fistula.
B   Tracheomalacia.
C   Cardiac anomalies.
D   Renal anomalies.
E   Imperforate anus.

16.7   Congenital hypertrophic pyloric stenosis:
A   Often manifests at birth.
B   May show visible peristalsis.
C   Is caused by thickening of the circular layer of muscle.
D   May cause altered blood gases because of vomiting.
E   Is cured by pyloromyotomy.

(Answers overleaf)

16.4	A	False	It is a multicystic swelling derived from persistent primitive lymph sacs. It is a lymphangioma.
	B	False	Dermoid cysts are due to failure of fusion of sections of the embryo. They are usually seen in the midline of the neck, lateral angle of the eye and behind the pinna of the ear.
	C	True	
	D	True	It may also extend into the thorax.
	E	False	There is a minimal degree of spontaneous resolution, but often excision is required. An MRI scan is indicated to outline the extent of the lesion.

16.5	A	False	The septum transversum contributes to the central tendon of the diaphragm.
	B	False	It contributes to the crura and the parts adjacent to the vertebral column.
	C	True	On the ipsilateral side, the presence of abdominal contents prevents normal development of the lung. Associated mediastinal shift will cause hypoplasia of the contralateral lung.
	D	True	This is due to a defect in the formation of the pleuroperitoneal membrane closing the pleuroperitoneal canal. It is more common on the left side as this side closes last.
	E	True	These are small hernias and only rarely associated with lung hypoplasia. However, these too require surgical repair.

16.6	A	True	
	B	True	
	C	True	
	D	True	
	E	True	

16.7	A	False	It usually manifests 3–5 weeks after birth.
	B	True	Also, there may be a palpable lump in the right hypochondrium.
	C	True	
	D	True	The baby is dehydrated, hypochloraemic and alkalotic.
	E	True	In pyloromyotomy the hypertrophied muscle is split without opening the mucosa.

16.8   Concerning duodenal atresia:
A   It is caused by vascular accident during the second trimester.
B   Obstruction commonly is in the first part of the duodenum.
C   Plain abdominal X-ray reveals a double bubble appearance.
D   It can be diagnosed antenatally.
E   Duodenoduodenostomy is the operation of choice.

16.9   Regarding rotation of the midgut:
A   It rotates through 90° clockwise while in the umbilical cord.
B   It rotates through 180° anticlockwise as the midgut returns to the abdomen during the 10th week.
C   In malrotation, plain X-ray shows small bowel on the left and large bowel on the right.
D   Malrotation can cause duodenal obstruction.
E   Malrotation may cause volvulus.

16.10 Regarding gastroschisis and exomphalos:
A   In gastroschisis the anterior abdominal wall is defective.
B   Exomphalos is a small umbilical hernia.
C   In gastroschisis the herniated contents are covered by a layer of amniotic membrane.
D   Exomphalos is rarely associated with other congenital anomalies.
E   Surgical closure of the anterior abdominal wall defect is curative in both conditions.

(Answers overleaf)

16.8 **A** **False** It occurs during the eighth week because of failure of recanalization of the developing duodenum. Small bowel (jejunal and ileal) and large bowel atresias occur during fourth to sixth months (second trimester) owing to ischaemic vascular accident of the mesentery.

    B **False** The common site is just distal to the ampulla of Vater; vomitus is bile-stained.

    C **True** The first bubble is air in the distended stomach and the second is air in the distended duodenum.

    D **True** Antenatal scan may show a double cystic appearance due to swallowed amniotic fluid not being able to pass through the gut. It may lead to polyhydramnios.

    E **True** It is the most physiological correction; duodenojejunostomy leaves a blind loop.

16.9 **A** **False** The rotation at this stage is anticlockwise.

    B **True** The superior mesenteric artery acts as the axis for the rotation.

    C **False** Normal rotation brings the small bowel to the left and the large bowel to the right; the positions are reversed in malrotation.

    D **True** It is caused by fibrous bands stretching from the caecum across the duodenum.

    E **True** The base of the mesentery is narrow and is not fixed at either end. The gut twists on the superior mesenteric artery and becomes ischaemic causing the volvulus. The neonate/infant presents with bilious vomiting and an X-ray shows no gas distal to the stomach. This requires emergency laparotomy.

16.10 **A** **True** All the muscles are in existence, but there is a full-thickness defect usually adjacent to the right side of the umbilical cord.

    B **False** Umbilical hernias are covered by skin, whereas in exomphalos the covering is amniotic membrane.

    C **False** There is no covering in gastroschisis. The intestines are exposed to amniotic fluid which results in dismotile thickened bowel wall.

    D **False** Exomphalos is often associated with other major congenital anomalies. When detected antenatally, chromosomal analysis is recommended.

    E **False** Once the defect is closed the gut functions normally in exomphalos but may not do so in gastroschisis.

16.11   Meckel's diverticulum:
A   Is a persistent vitellointestinal duct.
B   Is present in 2% of the population.
C   May have a fistulous connection to the umbilicus.
D   May contain gastric mucosa.
E   Can be detected antenatally by ultrasound scans.

16.12   Regarding anorectal development and anomalies:
A   The cloacal membrane separates the cloaca into urinary and anorectal regions.
B   Muscles of the pelvic floor and sphincters develop from the urorectal septum.
C   A high anorectal anomaly is commonly associated with a fistula.
D   A low anorectal anomaly is associated with poor development of sphincter muscles.
E   A pull-through operation to correct a high lesion is done only when the baby is a few months old.

16.13   Regarding Hirschsprung's disease:
A   It is caused by aganglionosis of a segment of the colon.
B   It commonly affects the rectosigmoid region.
C   Nerve fibres are absent in the segment affected.
D   Babies affected fail to pass meconium.
E   It may be familial.

(Answers overleaf)

16.11 A   True   The vitellointestinal duct connects the midgut to the yolk sac.

  B   True   It is located in the ileum 2 feet (60 cm) away from the ileocaecal valve and it is 2 inches (5 cm) long.

  C   True   It can present also as a swelling at the umbilicus, or as an umbilical polyp.

  D   True   It may cause bleeding due to peptic ulceration of the ectopic gastric mucosa; the persistent fibrous bands extending to the umbilicus may cause intestinal obstruction and volvulus.

  E   False   It is difficult to detect even after birth. A radiolabelled technetium scan looking for ectopic gastric mucosa is positive in only 70% of patients with rectal bleeding due to Meckel's diverticulum.

16.12 A   False   The cloacal membrane separates the cloaca (from which the urinary passages and the anorectal region are developed) from the amniotic cavity.

  B   True   The urorectal septum separates the anorectal region from the urinary passages.

  C   True   The fistula is between the rectum and the bladder in the male and between the rectum and the vagina in the female. The fistula is due to poor development of the urorectal septum.

  D   False   Sphincters are mostly developed in a low lesion (unlike a high lesion). However, even these babies may have problems with continence.

  E   False   If the baby is healthy and if the surgeon is experienced it can be done earlier, otherwise a two-stage procedure is envisaged with a colostomy followed by a pull-through operation.

16.13 A   True   A segment of the colon is without the ganglionic cells of the myenteric plexus.

  B   True   This area is often affected, but aganglionosis may extend proximally as well.

  C   False   Nerve fibres are hypertrophied in the affected area and they can be stained for cholinesterase in biopsy specimens.

  D   True   The segment affected is functionally obstructed with no peristalsis. The part proximal to the obstruction distends to produce the megacolon. The abdomen is distended and the baby presents with bilious vomiting about 36 hours after birth.

  E   True   Occasionally more than one child is affected. There is still no gene probe to test for the condition antenatally.

16.14 Regarding urinary tract development and anomalies:
A The definitive kidneys initially develop in the pelvis.
B There is no surgical consequence associated with the congenital absence of one kidney.
C A horseshoe kidney may complicate surgery to the abdominal aorta.
D A pelvic kidney may cause a mass in the iliac fossa.
E The commonest site of unilateral ureteric obstruction of congenital origin is at its lower end.

16.15 Hypospadias:
A Is caused by failure of fusion of the urogenital folds forming the penis.
B Is one of the commonest congenital anomalies affecting boys.
C In the majority, will be glandular where the urethral opening is on the glans penis.
D May be associated with congenital hyperplasia of the adrenal glands.
E May be associated with intersex in severe cases.

16.16 Regarding hernias, hydrocele and undescended testis:
A An encysted hydrocele of the cord develops in the gubernaculum testis.
B Congenital hernia and congenital hydrocele are caused by a patent processus vaginalis.
C Ectopic testes are more common than undescended testis.
D There is a risk of testicular tumour developing in a child with undescended testis.
E There is a risk of developing infertility even after orchidopexy.

(Answers overleaf)

16.14 A **True** The nephrons develop from the metanephros and the collecting ducts; the calyces and the ureter from the ureteric bud of the mesonephric duct. The kidneys ascend gradually from the pelvis to their adult position.

B **False** The existing kidney can be obstructed causing anuria; it can be removed without it being realized that it is a solitary kidney.

C **True** It lies across the abdominal aorta.

D **True** It may ascend only up to the iliac fossa and may be felt as a mass. It may be solitary and removed in error. It may be prone to trauma.

E **False** The commonest site is the pelviureteric junction (PUJ). Obstruction can be due to ureteric kink, aberrant blood vessel, or an extrinsic band.

16.15 A **True**

B **True** It occurs in 3 per 1000 boys.

C **True** This is the minor variety; in the moderate type the urethra opens on the body of the penis (penile type) and in the severe variety it opens at the base of the penis or in the perineum (perineal).

D **True**

E **True** The individual may have XX chromosomes; the gonads may not be felt.

16.16 A **False** It develops in a partially obliterated processus vaginalis.

B **True** Herniation of abdominal contents into the processus produces a congenital inguinal hernia; fluid collection within the processus is called a congenital hydrocele.

C **False** Ectopic testes – where the testes descend to abnormal positions – are very uncommon. Ectopic testis may be found in the perineum, upper part of the femoral triangle, root of the penis and in the anterior abdominal wall.

D **True** The incidence is 1 in 70, whereas in the normal population it is 1 in 5000. The risk is proportional to the degree of maldescent. In unilateral cases there is a 25% chance of malignancy developing in the contralateral testis which is normally descended.

E **True** Bilateral undescended testes cause infertility if orchidopexy is not done. Even after orchidopexy there is a risk of infertility in 10–25% of cases. Orchidopexy before 2 years of age offers the best chance of fertility.

16.17 Regarding the fetal circulation:
A   The ligamentum teres is the remnant of the left umbilical vein.
B   Oxygenated blood runs from the placenta to the fetus via the umbilical arteries.
C   In utero, blood flows from the left to the right atrium via the foramen ovale.
D   The umbilical arteries arise from the iliac arteries.
E   The ductus arteriosus connects the pulmonary artery to the descending aorta.

16.18 Regarding fluid and electrolyte balance:
A   The percentage of body weight due to water is higher in premature babies.
B   Small babies need less fluid per kg than larger ones.
C   Relative to weight, babies require less potassium than adults.
D   Owing to the frailty of peripheral veins, 2.5% dextrose solutions should be the maximum strength used.
E   Neonates are at particular risk of becoming hypercalcaemic.

16.19 Neonates:
A   Will need parenteral nutrition after 2 days without feeding.
B   Have a different response to surgery which, unlike that of adults, leads to postoperative hypoglycaemia.
C   When septic, should not receive broad-spectrum antibiotics before culture results because of the development of resistance.
D   When ventilated, require less fluids than non-ventilated babies.
E   Must all have vitamin K preoperatively.

(Answers overleaf)

16.17 A True It runs in the falciform ligament of the liver.
     B False The umbilical arteries carry deoxygenated blood to the placenta.
     C False Blood flow is from the right to the left.
     D True
     E True

16.18 A True In a full-term neonate 75% of the body is water. In a 26-week neonate 86% is water.
     B False Owing to the larger surface area of small babies, insensible losses are greater.
     C False Babies require 2–3 mmol of potassium per kilogram, whereas adults only need 1 mmol/kg.
     D False Peripheral veins are much more tolerant of hypertonic solution, so 10% dextrose is always used.
     E False They can easily become hypocalcaemic and hypomagnesaemic so should have supplementation in maintenance fluids.

16.19 A True In comparison, premature babies will need parenteral nutrition only 1 day after cessation of feeding.
     B False The response mimics that of the adult with an increase in adrenaline and decrease in insulin leading to hyperglycaemia.
     C False Appropriate broad spectrum antibiotics should be given intravenously before culture results are available.
     D True Ventilated babies are still and so insensible losses are less.
     E True This is because blood clotting mechanisms are insufficiently developed.

17. Alimentary system

17.1 **With regard to abdominal incisions:**
- **A** The midline incision is made through the linea alba.
- **B** The seventh intercostal nerve is in danger in a subcostal incision.
- **C** The gridiron incision is made at McBurney's point.
- **D** Adherence of the posterior rectus sheath to the rectus abdominis is encountered in a paramedian incision.
- **E** A pararectus incision (Battle incision) is commonly used for appendicectomy.

17.2 **Concerning the inguinal canal:**
- **A** The deep inguinal ring is 1 cm above the midpoint of the inguinal ligament.
- **B** The superficial inguinal ring is reinforced posteriorly by the conjoint tendon.
- **C** Between the two inguinal rings the posterior wall consists of transversalis fascia only.
- **D** The iliohypogastric nerve passes through the canal.
- **E** The inferior epigastric artery is lateral to the deep ring.

17.3 **Regarding inguinal hernias:**
- **A** All inguinal hernias pass through the deep inguinal ring.
- **B** An indirect hernia passes lateral to the inferior epigastric artery.
- **C** An indirect hernia, if large, may reach the scrotum.
- **D** A direct hernia is within the coverings of the spermatic cord.
- **E** An indirect hernia may be of congenital origin.

17.1   **A**   **True**   It is an excellent incision for routine and rapid access to the peritoneal cavity.

       B   **False**   A subcostal (Kocher's) incision is made about 2.5 cm below the costal margin. The nerve encountered is the ninth intercostal nerve, damage to which may weaken the rectus abdominis.

       C   **True**   McBurney's point is two-thirds of the way down a line connecting the umbilicus to the anterior superior iliac spine.

       D   **False**   The anterior wall of the rectus sheath is adherent to the tendinous intersections of the rectus and has to be dissected off. The posterior rectus sheath is not adherent to the muscle.

       E   **False**   A gridiron incision is more commonly used for appendicectomy. A pararectus incision is used to insert a Tenckhoff catheter for ambulatory peritoneal dialysis.

17.2   **A**   **True**   This is just lateral to the midinguinal point which is halfway between the anterior superior iliac spine and the pubic symphysis.

       B   **True**   The conjoint tendon reinforcing the posterior wall helps to offset the weakness of the anterior wall produced by the superficial ring.

       C   **False**   The medial part of the posterior wall is formed by the conjoint tendon as well.

       D   **False**   It transmits the spermatic cord and the ilioinguinal nerve in the male and the round ligament of the uterus and the ilioinguinal nerve in the female.

       E   **False**   The artery is medial to the deep ring.

17.3   **A**   **False**   Indirect hernias pass though the deep ring. Direct hernias invaginate the posterior wall of the inguinal canal.

       B   **True**   The deep ring, through which it passes, is lateral to the artery.

       C   **True**   As the hernia is within the coverings of the spermatic cord there is nothing blocking it from doing so.

       D   **False**   A direct hernia is separate from the cord as it bulges directly through the posterior wall of the canal medial to the inferior epigastric artery.

       E   **True**   If the processus vaginalis is not obliterated, it can contain a congenital hernia.

17.4   The femoral canal:
   A   Contains the femoral artery and vein.
   B   Transmits the long saphenous vein.
   C   Contains the superficial inguinal lymph nodes.
   D   Has its lateral boundary formed by the lacunar ligament.
   E   Is larger in the female.

17.5   Regarding the peritoneal ligaments and spaces:
   A   The falciform ligament contains the obliterated umbilical artery.
   B   The median umbilical ligament is formed by the obliterated urachus.
   C   The epiploic foramen is bounded anteriorly by the free border of the lesser omentum.
   D   The right and left subphrenic spaces are separated by the coronary ligament.
   E   The gastrosplenic and the lienorenal ligaments form the left boundary of the lesser sac.

(Answers overleaf)

17.4 **A** **False** The femoral sheath contains the femoral artery and vein and medial to the vein the femoral canal.

B **False** The long saphenous vein passes through the saphenous opening to join the femoral vein.

C **False** The femoral canal has Cloquet's node which is one of the deep inguinal nodes. The superficial inguinal nodes are superficial to the deep fascia.

D **False** The canal is bounded laterally by the femoral vein. The lacunar ligament is the medial boundary of the femoral ring which is the upper opening of the canal. The femoral ring is narrow and its boundaries are unyielding, hence femoral hernias are commonly irreducible and are prone to strangulation.

E **True** This is because the female pelvis is wider; femoral hernias are more common in the female.

17.5 **A** **False** It contains the obliterated umbilical vein. The obliterated umbilical arteries form the lateral umbilical ligaments in the lower part of the anterior abdominal wall.

B **True** It extends from the bladder to the umbilicus.

C **True** The anterior boundary is the free border of the lesser omentum, which contains the hepatic artery, bile duct and the portal vein. If the cystic artery is torn during cholecystectomy, the hepatic artery can be compressed between finger and thumb at this level. This is known as Pringle's manoeuvre.

D **False** The spaces are on either side of the falciform ligament. The coronary ligament and the liver form the upper boundary of the right subhepatic space (pouch of Rutherford Morrison). This is the most dependent part of the peritoneal cavity in the recumbent position, and hence is a potential site for subphrenic abscess formation from perforated peptic ulcer, perforated appendicitis, or perforated diverticulitis.

E **True** They form the boundary along with the spleen.

17.6   Regarding the oesophagus:
A   It is approximately 25 cm long in the adult.
B   The cervical part is related to both the recurrent laryngeal nerves.
C   The thoracic part is closely related to the aorta.
D   It has a narrowing at the diaphragmatic hiatus.
E   Its mucous membrane contains stratified squamous epithelium.

17.7   At the pyloric region of the stomach:
A   The pyloric sphincter is seen and felt at operation.
B   The prepyloric vein helps the surgeon to identify the pylorus.
C   The pylorus always lies at the transpyloric plane.
D   The lymphatic drainage is to the subpyloric nodes.
E   Gastric glands predominantly contain parietal and chief cells.

17.8   The duodenum:
A   Is retroperitoneal throughout.
B   Develops from the foregut and midgut.
C   Has the gastroduodenal artery lying anteriorly to its first part.
D   Has its second part situated behind the hilum of the right kidney.
E   Has the opening of the bile duct and the pancreatic duct on the major duodenal papilla.

(Answers overleaf)

17.6   **A**   **True**   It extends from the lower border of the cricoid to the cardiac orifice of the stomach.

    B   **True**   The nerves lie in the groove between the trachea and the oesophagus on either side.

    C   **True**   The arch of the aorta is on its left side. The descending thoracic aorta is closely related to it on its left side except in the lower part where the oesophagus crosses in front of the aorta to lie on its left side.

    D   **True**   It also has narrowings at its commencement and where it is crossed by the left bronchus.

    E   **True**   Occasionally there may be gastric mucosa in the lower part of the oesophagus.

17.7   **A**   **True**   It is a prominent anatomical sphincter formed by thickening of the circular muscle.

    B   **True**   The vein is constant and crosses the anterior surface of the pylorus, running vertically downwards.

    C   **False**   It is completely invested with peritoneum, is mobile and the position is variable.

    D   **True**   The region drains to the subpyloric nodes and then to the coeliac nodes. In carcinoma of the stomach, retrograde spread may occur into the lymph nodes at the porta hepatis causing compression of the bile ducts and obstructive jaundice.

    E   **False**   The gastric glands here contain mostly mucous cells. There are also gastrin-producing G cells. Chief cells and parietal cells are mostly in the fundus and the body of the stomach.

17.8   **A**   **False**   The first inch is completely covered by peritoneum.

    B   **True**   The point of entry of the bile duct and the pancreatic duct marks the junction between the foregut and midgut.

    C   **False**   The gastroduodenal artery lies posteriorly. Bleeding from this vessel is a complication of a duodenal ulcer on the posterior wall.

    D   **False**   The hilum of the right kidney and the ureter lie posteriorly.

    E   **True**   This point is about 10 cm distal to the pylorus on the posteromedial wall of the second part of the duodenum.

17.9 Regarding the jejunum and ileum:
 A   The ileum has a thicker wall.
 B   The jejunum is of greater diameter than the ileum.
 C   In general, the jejunum is more likely to be found at or above the level of the umbilicus.
 D   There are more arterial arcades in the jejunal mesentery.
 E   Peyer's patches are present in the jejunal mucosa.

17.10 Regarding Meckel's diverticulum (ileal diverticulum):
 A   It represents the remains of the urachus.
 B   It is usually situated at the junction between the jejunum and ileum.
 C   Inflammation causes pain in the right iliac fossa.
 D   It may be attached to the umbilicus.
 E   It may contain gastric mucosa.

17.11 With regard to the appendix:
 A   The surface marking is at McBurney's point.
 B   The position of the base is inconstant.
 C   The tip lies most commonly in the retrocaecal position.
 D   It has a mesentery.
 E   The appendicular artery is functionally an end artery.

17.12 Regarding the sigmoid colon:
 A   It has a mesentery.
 B   There are no taeniae coli.
 C   Appendices epiploicae are less numerous than in the rest of the colon.
 D   It is related to the bladder in the male.
 E   The marginal artery (of Drummond) is weakest at the rectosigmoid junction.

(Answers overleaf)

17.9 **A** **False** The jejunal wall is thicker owing to circular folds or plicae circularis.
B **True** Normally it also has larger villi in the mucosa.
C **True** However, the position is variable as the small gut is mobile.
D **False** The ileal arcades are more numerous with the terminal arteries short and straight.
E **False** Lymphoid accumulation increases in the distal part of the small gut. Peyer's patches are in the ileum.

17.10 **A** **False** It is the remnant of the vitelline duct.
B **False** It is found in the ileum about 2 feet from the ileocaecal valve.
C **True** It may mimic appendicitis.
D **True** It may be joined to the umbilicus by a fibrous cord and may cause volvulus.
E **True** Also, it may occasionally contain pancreatic mucosa. Either causes bleeding and even perforation.

17.11 **A** **True** This is two-thirds of the way down a line connecting the umbilicus to the anterior superior iliac spine.
B **False** The base has a constant position and is on the posteromedial wall of the caecum where the three taenia coli meet.
C **True** In about 75% of cases it lies behind the caecum.
D **True** It is triangular, descends behind the ileum and has the appendicular artery in its free border.
E **True** In acute appendicitis, its thrombosis causes gangrene and perforation.

17.12 **A** **True** The root of the sigmoid mesocolon has an inverted V-shaped attachment with its apex at the bifurcation of the left common iliac artery. The left ureter crosses this point.
B **False** Taeniae coli extend up to the rectosigmoid junction.
C **False** They are more numerous.
D **True** It is also related to the vagina in the female. Vesicocolic and vaginocolic fistulae can develop in diverticular diseases.
E **False** The weakest point is where the middle colic artery anastomoses with the left colic just proximal to the left colic flexure. Diminution of blood supply in this region may cause ischaemic colitis.

17.13 Regarding the rectum:
  A   The rectal ampulla is in the upper part.
  B   Waldeyer's fascia is in front of it.
  C   The sacral plexus is behind it.
  D   It is supplied by the inferior rectal artery.
  E   Mucosa is supplied by the middle rectal artery.

17.14 Regarding the anal canal:
  A   The upper half is derived from endoderm.
  B   It is lined throughout by columnar epithelium.
  C   It is insensitive to pain.
  D   It is surrounded by an involuntary external sphincter.
  E   The internal sphincter is continuous with the circular muscle of the rectum.

17.15 The levator ani:
  A   Originates mainly from the pelvic brim.
  B   Has the puboprostatae, pubovaginalis and puborectalis as its various parts.
  C   Is supplied by the ilioinguinal nerve.
  D   Contracts on coughing.
  E   Divides the superficial perineal pouch from the deep pouch.

(Answers overleaf)

17.13 A False The ampulla is in the lower part just above the pelvic floor.

B False Waldeyer's fascia is the condensation of pelvic fascia anchoring the rectum to the sacrum. Denonvilliers' fascia lies in front of the rectum separating it from the prostate (male) and the vagina (female). It is the plane of dissection in abdominoperineal excision of rectum.

C True This may be invaded by rectal cancer spreading posteriorly, causing sciatic pain.

D False The superior rectal and middle rectal arteries supply the rectum. The inferior rectal artery supplies the lower anal canal.

E False The artery, which lies behind the rectum, is small and it supplies the musculature.

17.14 A True The lower half is from ectoderm; the junction between the two parts is where the anal valves (of Ball) are present. The anal valves connect the lower ends of the anal columns (columns of Morgagni).

B False The lower half derived from ectoderm is lined by stratified squamous epithelium. Consequently, carcinoma of the upper anal canal is an adenocarcinoma and that of the lower part is squamous cell carcinoma.

C False The lower half has a somatic supply and is very sensitive to pain.

D False The external sphincter is voluntary and has subcutaneous, superficial and deep parts. The deep part blends with the internal sphincter and the puborectalis part of the levator ani to form the anorectal ring, which is palpable on rectal examination. It maintains the angle between the rectum and anal canal.

E True

17.15 A False It originates from the back of the body of the pubis, the spine of the ischium, and between these from the fascia covering the obturator internus muscle.

B True The pubovaginalis and puboprostatae are attached to the perineal body and support it. The puborectalis winds round the anorectal junction and contributes to the anorectal ring.

C False On the pelvic surface it is supplied by a branch of S4 and on the perineal surface by the inferior rectal nerve and perineal branch of the pudendal nerve.

D True It opposes the downward pressure of the abdominal muscles and increases the intra-abdominal pressure.

E False The levator ani separates the pelvis from the perineum. The two perineal pouches are separated by the perineal membrane.

17.16   Regarding the mechanism of swallowing:
    A   Tactile receptors in the pharynx initiate the swallowing reflex.
    B   The palatopharyngeal folds move inwards.
    C   The vocal cords remain stationary.
    D   A lesion affecting the vagus nerves will abolish primary peristalsis in the oesophagus.
    E   Distension of the oesophagus initiates the primary peristalsis.

17.17   The lower oesophageal sphincter:
    A   Is at the cardio-oesophageal junction.
    B   Has subatmospheric pressure in between swallowing.
    C   Is a thickening of the circular muscle.
    D   Is innervated directly by the vagus nerve.
    E   Is caused to contract by gastrin.

17.18   During the gastric phase of acid secretion:
    A   Acetylcholine directly stimulates the parietal cells.
    B   Histamine potentiates the effect of gastrin on the parietal cells.
    C   Distension of the body and antrum acts as mechanical stimulation.
    D   Digested proteins directly stimulate the parietal cells.
    E   Alcohol inhibits acid release.

(Answers overleaf)

17.16 A True   Impulses are transmitted to the swallowing centre in the medulla by V, IX and X cranial nerves from where efferent impulses are transmitted through V, VII, X, and XII nerves to the muscles involved.

B True   The soft palate is raised and approximated on to this ridge to shut off the nasopharynx.

C False   The vocal cords are adducted. The inlet of the larynx is shut by raising the larynx and approximating it against the epiglottis.

D True   The impulses for the primary peristalsis in the oesophagus during swallowing are initiated at the centre in the medulla and are transmitted from the nucleus ambiguus through the vagus nerve.

E False   Distension of the oesophagus initiates the secondary peristalsis.

17.17 A False   It is the lower 4 cm of the oesophagus, half of it above the diaphragm and half below.

B False   The rest of the thoracic oesophagus has subatmospheric pressure during swallowing. The lower oesophageal sphincter is a high-pressure zone where the pressure averages 15–25 mmHg.

C False   There is no anatomical modification.

D False   It is innervated by the vagus through interneurons and the myenteric plexus.

E True

17.18 A True   Parietal cells have receptors for acetylcholine, gastrin and histamine.

B True   Histamine is the most powerful stimulant and it potentiates the action of gastrin and acetylcholine.

C True   Distension of the body excites vagal reflexes and that of the antrum will increase gastrin release through intramural cholinergic reflexes.

D False   Amino acids in the antrum stimulate the G cells to release gastrin and this in turn stimulates the parietal cells to release acid.

E False   Alcohol is a stimulant for gastric secretion.

17.19 Regarding gastrointestinal hormones:
A   They are released into the lumen of the gastrointestinal tract.
B   They are destroyed in their passage through the liver.
C   Gastrin release is inhibited by increased acid production.
D   Cholecystokinin (CCK) hastens gastric emptying.
E   Secretin stimulates an enzyme-rich secretion from the pancreas.

17.20 In a high-output fistula:
A   Up to 1500 ml of fluid is lost per day.
B   Nutrients are not lost.
C   The fistula behaves like an ileostomy.
D   Acidosis may result.
E   If the fistula is external, there will be excoriation of the skin.

17.21 Propulsion of colonic contents depends on:
A   Retrograde peristalsis.
B   Segmentation.
C   Mass movement.
D   Migrating motility complex.
E   Emotional states.

(Answers overleaf)

17.19 A False Like all other hormones they are released into the bloodstream.

B False Hormones pass through the liver unaltered to reach the target tissues.

C True It is also inhibited by secretin and somatostatin.

D False CCK delays gastric emptying. It causes contraction of the gall bladder and relaxation of the sphincter of Oddi in addition to stimulating the acinar cells of the pancreas to produce an enzyme-rich secretion.

E False It stimulates the duct cells of the pancreas to increase secretion of water and HCO_3^-.

17.20 A False The output is larger – up to 3–4 litres. The fluid lost is isotonic. The output in a low-output fistula is about 1500 ml.

B False Nutrients taken orally do not get absorbed and pass through the fistula virtually unchanged. Total parenteral feeding and replacement of fluid and electrolytes are required.

C False The low-output fistula behaves like an ileostomy. High-output fistulas occur in the upper small bowel, whereas low-output fistulas are in the ileum.

D True This is due to loss of pancreatic juice and bile, both of which are alkaline.

E True This is due to digestive enzymes (trypsin) in the pancreatic secretion. Skin protection is required.

17.21 A True This is also known as antiperistalsis and is characterized by annular contractions moving in the direction opposite to that of the contents. It occurs chiefly in the ascending colon.

B True In this, occurring mostly in the transverse and descending colon, contraction rings of about 2.5 cm long appear, dividing the bowel into segments. The region in between contraction rings is relaxed.

C True This occurs two to three times a day and is initiated by a gastrocolic reflex caused by food entering the stomach. These are strong peristaltic waves covering long distances in the transverse and descending colon.

D False The migrating motility complex moves contents in the small intestine.

E True Colonic movements are affected by emotional state and also physical activity. Transit times are increased by high-fibre content of the diet.

17.22 Regarding bile pigments and bile salts:
 A Biliverdin is reabsorbed in the distal ileum.
 B Lecithin increases the amount of bile salt that can be solubilized.
 C Secondary bile salts are produced in the liver.
 D Bile salt concentration of hepatic bile will be higher than that of gall bladder bile.
 E More than 80% of bile salts are absorbed into the portal circulation in the distal ileum.

17.23 Regarding detoxification and inactivation of drugs by the liver:
 A The process is performed by Kupffer cells.
 B Solubility of the drug is increased during the process.
 C The cytochrome P450 system accelerates the process.
 D Barbiturates inhibit the process.
 E Rifampicin accelerates detoxification of cyclosporin and warfarin.

17.24 Concerning a pancreatic fistula:
 A The amount of fluid lost is not a major problem.
 B Fluid lost is hypotonic.
 C It may cause acidosis.
 D The enzymes leaking out always cause digestion of skin.
 E Somatostatin is useful in drying up the fistula.

(Answers overleaf)

17.22 A **False** Biliverdin is formed by the breakdown of red cells. It is then reduced to bilirubin. Bilirubin is conjugated in the liver and excreted into the small intestine via the gall bladder and the bile duct. In the intestine, bilirubin is reduced to urobilinogen most of which is reabsorbed into blood and transported back to the liver for recirculation.

B **True** If more cholesterol is present in the bile than can be solubilized, cholesterol can crystallize to form gallstones.

C **False** Primary bile salts are formed in the liver from cholesterol by the hepatocytes. The colonic bacteria convert these to secondary bile salts.

D **False** The concentration is higher in gall bladder bile as the gall bladder concentrates bile by absorbing water along with Na^+, Cl^- and HCO_3^-.

E **True** The rest enters the colon to be converted to secondary bile salts, part of which is reabsorbed and the rest excreted in the faeces.

17.23 A **False** These are major liver functions and are performed by the hepatocytes.

B **True** Drug solubility is increased during the process. In phase 1 this is the major factor and the levels are brought down by increasing excretion.

C **True** Levels of phenytoin, warfarin, halothane, indomethacin and cyclosporin are reduced by this system.

D **False** Barbiturates increase the activity of cytochrome P450.

E **True** Rifampicin potentiates cytochrome P450.

17.24 A **False** The amount of fluid lost is considerable – up to 1–2 litres.

B **False** The fluid is isotonic and its loss in such high quantity will cause dehydration.

C **True** The pancreatic juice is alkaline, contains bicarbonate, and its loss causes acidosis.

D **False** The enzymes are in the inactive form when they are secreted by the pancreas and hence need not digest the skin. However, they can be activated by secondary infection.

E **True** Somatostatin is an inhibitory peptide, inhibiting pancreatic secretion.

17.25 Regarding mechanical disorders of the oesophagus:
  A   Sliding hernias are less common than rolling hernias.
  B   In rolling hernias, the cardio-oesophageal junction is lifted up into the thorax.
  C   In rolling hernias, the fundus may get incarcerated and strangulation may occur.
  D   In achalasia, the myenteric plexus is without nerve fibres in the affected segment.
  E   Dysphagia is worse for liquids than for solids.

17.26 Carcinoma of the oesophagus:
  A   Is reducing in incidence world-wide.
  B   Is associated with achalasia.
  C   Is most commonly adenocarcinoma.
  D   Spreads through the lymphatics.
  E   Is resectable at the time of diagnosis in the great majority.

17.27 Carcinoma of the stomach:
  A   Has a 90% survival rate after radical surgery if the tumour is confined to mucosa and submucosa.
  B   Is commonly associated with duodenal ulcer.
  C   Is adenocarcinoma in the intestinal type, squamous in the diffuse type.
  D   Can cause obstructive jaundice.
  E   May spread to ovary.

(Answers overleaf)

17.25 A   False   Sliding hernias are more common. Obesity and raised intra-abdominal pressure are contributory factors.

B   False   This happens in sliding hernias. However, in rolling hernias the fundus of the stomach rolls into the thorax and lies along the lower part of the oesophagus.

C   True   The fundus may press on the oesophagus causing obstruction. After strangulation it can perforate.

D   False   In achalasia, the ganglion cells in the myenteric plexus are missing in the affected segment.

E   True   Solids may press on the narrow area and expand it.

17.26 A   False   The incidence is increasing and there is considerable geographical variation. The incidence is very high in Iran where the condition is 300 times more common than in the UK. It is also common in North China.

B   True   Conditions producing stasis will increase the risk; there is a 22-fold increase with lye strictures, ninefold increase with oesophageal webs, sevenfold increase with achalasia and a sixfold increase in peptic strictures.

C   False   Most are squamous cell carcinomas; adenocarcinomas are seen towards the lower third. About 50% occur in the middle third of the oesophagus, 10–15% in the upper third and the rest in the lower third.

D   True   This occurs early. It can also spread through blood. Direct spread may cause tracheo-oesophageal fistula, as well as invasion into the aorta causing fatal haemorrhage.

E   False   Surgical resection is possible only in about 30–40% as the tumour would have spread into the adjoining organs at the time of diagnosis. The 5-year survival rate is only 5%.

17.27 A   True   However, it is still the second most common fatal malignancy, the first being carcinoma of the lung.

B   False   Occasionally it can be associated with gastric ulcers, but not with duodenal ulcer.

C   False   Almost all gastric carcinomas are adenocarcinomas; they are further classified as the intestinal type which has well-defined borders and the diffuse type which is more malignant.

D   True   This occurs because of retrograde spread to the lymph nodes at the porta hepatis.

E   True   They are known as Krukenberg tumours of the ovary.

17.28 Regarding Crohn's disease:
- **A** It affects only the ileum.
- **B** It may be caused by a genetic defect.
- **C** Lesions may mimic tuberculosis.
- **D** Investigation by barium enema will show Cantor's 'string' sign.
- **E** It is commonly complicated by fistula formation.

17.29 Regarding ulcerative colitis:
- **A** It most often affects the caecum.
- **B** It occasionally affects the terminal ileum.
- **C** It may be associated with ankylosing spondylitis.
- **D** Inflammation is confined to the mucosa.
- **E** It is associated with increased risk of developing colonic carcinoma.

17.30 Diverticular disease:
- **A** Is most commonly situated in the sigmoid colon.
- **B** Is caused by a high-fibre diet.
- **C** Is associated with atrophy of colonic muscle wall.
- **D** May cause colovesical fistula.
- **E** Is associated with increased risk of developing colonic carcinoma.

(Answers overleaf)

17.28 A False Most commonly it occurs in the ileum; however, no part of the gastrointestinal tract is exempt.

B True There is a strong family history in about 15–20% of patients. Genes coding for HLA antigens are more common in patients with Crohn's disease than in normal controls.

C True Both are granulomatous lesions. However, pale tubercles may be seen in the serosa in tuberculosis.

D True This is due to fibrosis and narrowing of the bowel lumen. Only a very narrow column of barium will pass through the affected area.

E True This is a common complication and may lead on to enterocutaneous fistula after surgery.

17.29 A False Rectum and sigmoid colon are affected most commonly, but it can extend to involve the whole colon.

B True Occasionally the last few centimetres of the ileum are ulcerated. It is known as 'backwash' ileitis.

C True There is association with conditions which have genetic predisposition, such as ankylosing spondylitis and sclerosing cholangitis.

D True Only in very severe cases are the muscle layers affected. This is unlike what happens in Crohn's disease where transmural inflammation is a feature.

E True The overall incidence is about 2%. However, in patients who have had the disease for 25 years it rises to 10%.

17.30 A True Intraluminal pressure here is higher than in the rest of the colon as the pressure is inversely proportional to the radius (Laplace's law).

B False Diverticulosis is rare in people who take a high-fibre diet.

C False The muscle wall is thickened and shortened. The hypertrophy is caused by a low-fibre diet and consequent small hard stool.

D True This is caused by inflammation and perforation which can also result in peritonitis, vaginocolic fistula and ileocolic fistula.

E False

17.31 The following colorectal polyps may become malignant:
A   Adenoma.
B   Hamartoma.
C   Metaplastic polyps.
D   Familial polyposis coli.
E   Juvenile polyp.

17.32 Regarding colorectal cancer:
A   Adenomas are precursors of most.
B   It is commoner in the transverse colon than in the rectum.
C   Oncogenes frequently altered are c-Ki-*ras* and c-*myc*.
D   There is a greater risk of ulcerative colitis developing into carcinoma than there is of Crohn's disease.
E   In Dukes' grade A, 5-year survival is 30%.

17.33 Regarding carcinoma of the anal canal:
A   Squamous cell carcinoma arises above the dentate line.
B   Basal cell carcinomas arise in the transitional zone.
C   It rarely spreads to inguinal lymph nodes.
D   Malignant melanomas spread to liver and lungs.
E   Squamous cell carcinomas are radiosensitive.

17.34 Regarding post-hepatic jaundice:
A   It is milder than prehepatic (haemolytic) jaundice.
B   Urine colour is normal.
C   Serum transaminase is grossly increased.
D   Serum alkaline phosphatase is elevated.
E   It may occasionally follow cholecystectomy.

(Answers overleaf)

17.31 **A** **True** Adenomas may give rise to adenocarcinoma.
B **False** Hamartomas are rare. They do not become malignant.
C **False** These are not neoplastic and therefore do not become malignant.
D **True** Cancer develops before the age of 40 in almost all untreated patients.
E **False** Juvenile polyp is a solitary hamartoma.

17.32 **A** **True** Adenomas develop in the colon during the second and third decades and malignant changes occur by the age of 40.
B **False** Only 10% of tumours are in the transverse colon whereas the rectum is affected in 30% of cases, the ascending colon being the next most frequent site (25%).
C **True** Loss or suppression of the tumour suppressor genes may also occur.
D **True** Frequent colonoscopy is required to detect early malignant changes.
E **False** Grade A is confined to the mucosa and muscularis mucosa but has not involved the muscularis externa, the main muscle layer. The survival rate at this stage is about 90%.

17.33 **A** **False** It arises below the dentate line and can extend upwards into the rectum and outwards to involve the sphincters.
B **True** The adenocarcinomas arise above the dentate line.
C **False** Those arising below the dentate line spread to the inguinal nodes initially, whereas adenocarcinomas (starting above the dentate line) primarily spread to the pelvic lymph nodes but can spread to the inguinal nodes if the tumour extends below the dentate line.
D **True** They do so when they spread through the bloodstream.
E **True** Basal cell carcinomas are also radiosensitive.

17.34 **A** **False** In prehepatic jaundice the jaundice is usually mild, whereas in post-hepatic jaundice it is often deep.
B **False** Urine colour is dark.
C **False** It is normal. Serum transaminase is elevated in hepatic jaundice.
D **True** It is grossly elevated.
E **True** This is due to stricture of the bile duct.

17.35 Hepatocellular carcinoma:
A Is commoner in the UK than in the Far East.
B Is associated with cirrhosis.
C Has α-fetoprotein in the blood as a diagnostic marker.
D Spreads through intrahepatic veins.
E Has a poor prognosis.

17.36 Regarding gallstones:
A Most are visible on plain X-ray.
B Pure cholesterol stones form less than 10% of stones.
C Oestrogen facilitates the chance of stone formation.
D Clofibrate, a cholesterol-lowering agent, inhibits stone formation.
E Bile pigment stones are formed from conjugated bilirubin.

17.37 Regarding chronic cholecystitis:
A It is usually associated with gallstones.
B It is more common in females than in males.
C The gall bladder is often palpable.
D The gall bladder is distended and has a thin wall.
E Aschoff–Rokitansky sinuses are seen histologically.

17.38 Carcinoma of the gall bladder:
A Commonly occurs in the fourth decade of life.
B Most often is a squamous cell carcinoma.
C Is asymptomatic in the early stages.
D May cause obstructive jaundice.
E Has a poor prognosis.

(Answers overleaf)

17.35 A **False** It is commoner in Africa and the Far East. It is rare in the UK.
    B **True** Cirrhosis, irrespective of its cause, can lead on to liver cell carcinoma.
    C **True** α-fetoprotein is secreted into the blood by the tumour.
    D **True** It also spreads through the lymphatics; however, distant metastasis is uncommon.
    E **True** Most patients die within 6 months of diagnosis.

17.36 A **False** Only 10% of the stones contain calcium, making them visible on plain X-ray.
    B **True** They are usually solitary and have a characteristic radial arrangement of crystals on cross-section.
    C **True** Oestrogen increases hepatic synthesis of cholesterol which is excreted in the bile. Cholesterol stones are formed in bile saturated with cholesterol.
    D **False** It can cause stone formation as it facilitates excretion of cholesterol in the bile.
    E **False** Pigment stones contain a calcium salt of unconjugated bile.

17.37 A **True** It is almost always associated with gallstones.
    B **True** It is encountered three times more often in females than in males.
    C **False** It is fibrosed and contracted and is not palpable.
    D **False** The walls are fibrosed and rigid and the gall bladder is contracted.
    E **True** These are glandular outpouchings of the mucosa deep into the muscle layer.

17.38 A **False** It occurs in the elderly.
    B **False** Adenocarcinomas are more common.
    C **True** Tumour invades the liver and adjacent organs and is advanced at presentation.
    D **True** It may be caused by invasion of the bile duct by tumour or by metastasis in the lymph nodes at the porta hepatis.
    E **True** The tumour is rarely resectable at presentation and the 5-year survival rate is less than 1%.

17.39 Acute pancreatitis:
A   May be caused by regurgitation of bile into the pancreatic duct.
B   Can induce fat necrosis.
C   Has raised serum amylase as a diagnostic feature.
D   May cause hypercalcaemia.
E   May cause chronic pancreatitis.

17.40 Carcinoma of the pancreas:
A   Commonly occurs in the elderly.
B   Is increasing in incidence in the UK.
C   Is associated with a palpable gall bladder in all cases.
D   Commonly spreads locally in the early stages.
E   Has a poor prognosis.

(Answers overleaf)

17.39 A True This can be caused by obstruction of the pancreatic duct at the ampulla of Vater. Increased ductal pressure will damage the acini causing leakage of enzymes into the pancreas.

  B True This is caused by lipase causing yellowish-white specks on the pancreas and adjoining fat-containing tissues.

  C True Serum amylase is raised in the acute phase, in 24–48 hours, but falls to normal later.

  D False Fat necrosis causes hypocalcaemia.

  E True Repeated attacks of acute pancreatitis can cause chronic pancreatitis.

17.40 A False The peak incidence is in the fifth and sixth decades.

  B True The incidence is also increasing in many other countries.

  C False Tumour in the head of the pancreas causes obstructive jaundice making the gall bladder palpable. Tumour elsewhere in the pancreas is symptomless until it is advanced.

  D True It spreads to adjacent structures, lymph nodes and liver; and also into the peritoneum and lungs.

  E True The tumour is symptomless in the early stages. The 5-year survival rate is less than 10%.

18. Genitourinary system

18.1 Regarding the anatomy of the kidneys:
A The hilums of both kidneys lie roughly at the transpyloric plane.
B The pelvis of the ureter lies anteriorly at the hilum.
C More than one renal artery may enter the kidney.
D There is perirenal fat inside the renal fascia.
E They are related to the pleural cavities separated by the diaphragm.

18.2 The ureter:
A Has a constriction at the pelviureteric junction.
B Is supplied throughout by branches from the renal artery.
C Has pacemakers in its pelvis regulating peristalsis.
D Has segmental innervation by L5–S1.
E And gonadal vein can be confused at operation, the vein being mistaken for the ureter.

(Answers overleaf)

18.1 **A** **True** The right kidney is slightly lower than the left.
B **False** The pelvis of the ureter is posterior at the hilum. The hilum contains, from anterior to posterior, the renal vein, the renal artery and the pelvis.
C **True** There can be accessory arteries. The renal artery divides into 3–5 segmental branches which further divide into 6–10 lobar arteries, one for each pyramid and associated cortex.
D **True** There is also perirenal fat outside the renal fascia (Gerota's fascia). The adrenal gland is also inside the renal fascia but within a separate compartment.
E **True** The pleural cavities extend up to the 12th rib at the back. The 12th rib is related to both the kidneys.

18.2 **A** **True** There are also constrictions at the point where it crosses the bifurcation of the common iliac artery and in the intramural portion within the bladder wall. A renal calculus can be arrested at these levels as it descends down the ureter.
B **False** It has a segmental blood supply from the renal artery, gonadal artery, internal iliac and the inferior vesical arteries.
C **True** These generate impulses to produce the peristaltic waves. There are 3–5 peristaltic waves/minute down the ureter.
D **False** Sympathetic innervation is by T11–L1 and parasympathetic by S2–S4. It has a rich sensory innervation. Pain is referred to the T11–L1 area.
E **True** The ureter, though retroperitoneal, is adherent to the peritoneum and also demonstrates peristaltic waves. The vein can be mistaken for it and inadvertently mobilized and cut.

18.3   Regarding the urinary bladder:
A   It is superiorly related to the sigmoid colon.
B   The detrusor is predominantly innervated by the adrenergic nerves.
C   Parasympathetic innervation is through fibres from S2–S4 segments.
D   The arterial supply is by branches of the internal iliac arteries.
E   The lymphatics drain into the internal iliac nodes.

18.4   Regarding renal functions:
A   Glomerular filtration rate is 500 ml per minute.
B   Proximal tubules reabsorb 50% of glucose.
C   50% of sodium in the glomerular filtrate is reabsorbed in the renal tubules.
D   Antidiuretic hormone (ADH) facilitates water resorption in the loop of Henle.
E   Aldosterone increases K^+ secretion in the distal tubules.

(Answers overleaf)

18.3 **A** **True** Diverticular disease of the sigmoid can cause colovesical fistula. In the female, the uterus lies superior to the bladder. Posteriorly, lie the seminal vesicles and the ductus deferens in the male and the vagina and the supravaginal cervix in the female.

B **False** The trigone has many adrenergic nerve endings whereas the detrusor innervation is predominantly cholinergic. M_3 muscarinic receptors are predominant.

C **True** Sympathetics are derived from T11–L2. There is an autonomic plexus with a number of ganglia through which a variety of neurotransmitters, in addition to acetyl choline and noradrenaline, regulate bladder functions.

D **True** The superior and inferior vesicle arteries supply the bladder. The venous drainage is to the venous plexus at the base of the bladder and then to the internal iliac vein.

E **True** Drainage is to the internal iliac nodes and from them to the para-aortic nodes.

18.4 **A** **False** The filtration rate is 125 ml per minute. Approximately 650 ml of blood circulates through each kidney per minute. The renal blood flow is about 25% of the cardiac output.

B **False** Almost all the glucose in the glomerular filtrate is reabsorbed in the proximal tubule up to a plasma glucose concentration of 200 mg/dl, beyond which the glucose load exceeds the capacity for resorption.

C **False** More than 99% of the filtered Na^+ is reabsorbed, more than half of this in the proximal tubule. In the descending limb of the loop of Henle, sodium chloride and water are reabsorbed passively, whereas in the ascending limb, which is impermeable to water, as well as in the distal tubule and the collecting tubule, sodium is actively pumped out against a concentration gradient.

D **False** Permeability of the distal tubules and the collecting tubules is increased by ADH so that water moves from the tubular lumen into the medullary interstitium where the osmolarity is higher. Dehydration results in release of ADH, increasing the water resorption in the distal nephron.

E **True** Aldosterone enhances sodium resorption and potassium secretion (into the lumen) in the distal tubules and collecting ducts.

18.5   Regarding hormones of the kidney:
A   Angiotensinogen is produced by the juxtaglomerular cells.
B   Hyponatraemia causes increased production of renin.
C   Kallikrein produced in the distal nephron is a vasoconstrictor.
D   Erythropoietin produced by the kidney regulates the renal blood flow.
E   25-hydroxycholecalciferol is activated in the kidney.

18.6   In normal kidney function:
A   Approximately 10% of the cardiac output passes through the kidneys every minute.
B   Frusemide is a loop diuretic.
C   Sympathetic nerves cause release of renin from juxtaglomerular cells.
D   Renin acts on angiotensin I to convert it to angiotensin II.
E   Aldosterone is produced by the zona fasciculata of the adrenal gland.

18.7   Regarding acute renal failure:
A   Oliguria is a daily urine output of less than 200 ml.
B H_2-receptor antagonists are of use.
C   Increased excretion of potassium leads to hypokalaemia.
D   Diuresis following oliguresis indicates worsening of renal function.
E   Plain abdominal X-rays are of no value.

(Answers overleaf)

18.5 **A** **False** Angiotensinogen is produced in the liver and is converted to angiotensin I by renin produced in the kidney.

  B **True** Sympathetic stimulation and hyponatraemia stimulate the juxtaglomerular cells to produce renin. Renin converts angiotensinogen to angiotensin I, which is converted to angiotensin II by angiotensin-converting enzyme (ACE). Angiotensin II stimulates the zona glomerulosa to produce aldosterone, which in turn facilitates sodium resorption in the distal tubules and collecting ducts.

  C **False** It is a vasodilator.

  D **False** Hypoxia causes erythropoietin production in the kidney. It stimulates haemopoiesis and increases the reticulocyte count in the peripheral blood. Synthesized erythropoietin is used in treating anaemia associated with chronic renal failure.

  E **True** 1α-hydroxylase produced in the kidney converts 25-hydroxycholecalciferol into 1,25-dihydroxycholecalciferol which promotes calcium absorption in the gut.

18.6 **A** **False** The figure is closer to 25% of the cardiac output.

  B **True** It acts to inhibit chloride and sodium resorption from the descending limb.

  C **True** Sympathetic activity is in response to hyponatraemia and decreased afferent arteriolar pressure.

  D **False** Renin causes conversion of angiotensinogen to angiotensin I.

  E **False** It is produced in the zona glomerulosa and causes sodium resorption and vasoconstriction.

18.7 **A** **False** Oliguria is a daily urine output less than 500 ml per day or 20 ml per hour.

  B **True** There is an increased incidence of gastrointestinal bleeding.

  C **False** Hyperkalaemia is a common problem and can be an indication for dialysis.

  D **False** Diuresis occurs in the recovery period.

  E **False** They are useful for ascertaining postrenal causes.

18.8 **In chronic renal failure:**
A   The associated anaemia is hypochromic microcytic.
B   Oliguria is an early sign.
C   Dialysis is essential when the creatinine level rises above 500 mmol/l.
D   Urine output should be maintained at supranormal levels.
E   Metabolic acidosis is a common complication.

18.9 **Regarding investigations of the urinary tract:**
A   Approximately 1 g of protein is excreted in the urine in 24 hours.
B   Creatinine clearance is used to measure glomerular filtration rate.
C   Residual volumes above 150 ml suggest detrusor dysfunction.
D   The intravenous urogram is the gold-standard investigation in urinary tract obstruction.
E   Normal urine is alkaline.

18.10 **Regarding acute renal failure:**
A   Renal blood flow is reduced to 30–40% of normal.
B   It can be caused by bacterial endocarditis.
C   Fluid intake should be restricted to 500 ml per day.
D   Dialysis should be done in all cases.
E   It is a condition with a high mortality rate.

18.11 **Chronic renal failure:**
A   Can be caused by hypertension.
B   Can be associated with polycystic disease of the kidney.
C   Is associated with polyuria.
D   Causes anaemia.
E   May cause secondary hyperparathyroidism.

(Answers overleaf)

18.8 **A** **False** It is a normochromic normocytic anaemia.
     B **False** Patients lose the ability to concentrate the urine and therefore have polyuria.
     C **False** Dialysis is usually instituted at creatinine levels above 1000 mmol/l. Creatinine level is a good indicator of the severity of the problem.
     D **False** A daily output of 1000 ml is desirable.
     E **True** It is due to decreased ammonium ion excretion.

18.9 **A** **False** Excretion is usually less than 100 mg.
     B **True** It is normally 100–140 ml per minute.
     C **True** The best way of measuring detrusor function is simultaneous measurement of bladder and rectal pressures.
     D **True** However, ultrasound scans with KUB (kidneys, ureters and bladder) X-rays have a good pick-up rate and are non-invasive.
     E **False** Urine pH ranges between 4.5–8.0.

18.10 **A** **True** The glomerular filtration rate is reduced to about 5 ml per minute.
     B **True** Prerenal causes are circulatory collapse due to blood loss, trauma or septicaemia.
     C **True** 500 ml is the fluid loss other than through the kidney (insensible loss). This amount is usually given orally. Sodium intake also is restricted to 20–30 mmol per day.
     D **False** Dialysis is done in cases where conservative treatment fails.
     E **True** It is especially high in cases associated with haemorrhage, trauma, peritonitis, advanced age and infection.

18.11 **A** **True** The commonest causes are chronic glomerulonephritis and pyelonephritis. Approximately 10% of cases are due to hypertension producing nephrosclerosis.
     B **True** There is an association in about 5% of cases.
     C **True** The ability of the kidney to concentrate urine is lost. However, a third of patients with chronic retention of urine develop chronic renal failure.
     D **True** This is due to erythropoietin deficiency and can be treated with human synthetic erythropoietin.
     E **True** This is due to reduced serum calcium levels. It can cause osteomalacia which is resistant to vitamin D.

18.12 Urinary calculi:
A   Are more common in women than in men.
B   Are usually radio-opaque.
C   Are most commonly calcium oxalate stones.
D   If they are phosphate stones, give rise to staghorn calculus.
E   May cause hydronephrosis.

18.13 Hypernephroma (renal cell carcinoma or Grawitz's tumour):
A   Is the commonest abdominal malignancy in children.
B   Is associated with polycythaemia.
C   May extend into the left renal vein.
D   May cause haematuria.
E   May spread to lung.

18.14 Regarding urothelial tumours:
A   The majority occur in the urinary bladder.
B   They are associated with haematuria.
C   Carcinoma in situ is a benign condition which does not require proactive treatment.
D   Radical surgery is indicated in the early stages.
E   They tend to recur after resection.

(Answers overleaf)

18.12 A False They are five times more common in men than in women.
 B True 90% of urinary calculi are radio-opaque.
 C True 75% are oxalate stones. These have mulberry-shaped irregular surfaces and causes haematuria in the early stages. They occur in alkaline urine.
 D True They have smooth surfaces and can grow until they fill the calyces, taking their staghorn shape. 5% of stones are phosphate stones.
 E True Obstruction of the urinary tract can lead on to hydronephrosis.

18.13 A False Wilms' tumour is the commonest abdominal malignancy in children. Hypernephroma or renal adenocarcinoma occurs in the 40–70 age group. Men are affected more than women and the tumour may occur bilaterally.
 B True This is due to excess of erythropoietin production. It is also associated with hypertension due to excess of renin.
 C True The condition can present with left-sided varicocele.
 D True The tumour may invade the renal pelvis.
 E True It can spread through the blood to liver, lungs and bones. It gives rise to cannon ball metastases in the lung.

18.14 A True About 90% occur in the bladder, 9% in the renal pelvis and 1% in the ureter.
 B True Haematuria is a presenting feature. It is painless and in the early stages microscopic.
 C False Carcinoma in situ in the case of urothelial tumours needs early intervention as it develops into a poorly differentiated aggressive tumour.
 D True Urothelial tumours are aggressive and invasive and will require radical surgery at an early stage.
 E True In about 70% of cases the tumour recurs after endoscopic resection. Intravesical chemotherapy after resection may reduce recurrence.

18.15 Regarding the male urethra:
   A   It is divided into anterior and posterior urethra.
   B   The bladder neck sphincter prevents retrograde ejaculation.
   C   The distal urethral sphincter has a triple innervation.
   D   The lumen is uniform throughout.
   E   It is lined throughout by transitional epithelium.

18.16 Regarding posterior urethral injuries:
   A   They are often associated with pelvic fractures.
   B   The distal urethral sphincter is damaged.
   C   A catheter should be passed to empty the bladder.
   D   They may be caused by rupture of the bulbar urethra.
   E   Swelling within Buck's fascia is increased on voiding.

(Answers overleaf)

18.15 A True   The posterior urethra, 6 cm long, comprises the prostatic urethra (4 cm) and the membranous urethra (2 cm), the latter being surrounded by the distal sphincter mechanism. The anterior urethra is inside the corpus spongiosum of the penis and is further divided into bulbar and pendulous parts.

B True   It consists mostly of circular muscle fibres. This sphincter can help to maintain continence if the distal sphincter is destroyed.

C True   This sphincter consists of a lissosphincter (smooth muscle) and a rhabdosphincter (striated muscle) and is innervated by sympathetic, parasympathetic and somatic nerves.

D False   The prostatic urethra is the widest part of the urethra. There are dilatations in the bulbar region and also just before the external opening, the navicular fossa. The narrowest parts of the urethra are at the bladder neck, in the membranous part, just proximal to the navicular fossa and at the external meatus. The membranous urethra is the least dilatable part.

E False   The urethra is lined by transitional epithelium except for the navicular fossa and the external meatus.

18.16 A True   This is because the posterior urethra (prostatic urethra and membranous urethra) is closely related to the body of the pubis and the pubic rami. Injury can also be iatrogenic, namely during transurethral resection of the prostate (TURP).

B True   The injury is in the region of the sphincter.

C False   Passage of a catheter may convert an incomplete tear into a complete rupture.

D False   The bulbar and the rest of the penile urethra form the anterior urethra. The bulbar urethra can be injured by instrumentation or from a fall astride an object crushing the urethra against the pubic symphysis.

E False   Swelling and a haematoma within Buck's fascia is characteristic of an anterior urethral injury. However, it is increased during voiding as more urine is collected.

18.17 Regarding the prostate gland:
    A   The urethra passes through its middle.
    B   It contains no muscle fibres.
    C   It is surrounded by a venous plexus draining into the vertebral venous plexus.
    D   It has a posterior median groove that is felt on rectal examination.
    E   The median lobe lies between the ejaculatory duct and the urethra.

18.18 Regarding carcinoma of the prostate:
    A   It is usually a squamous cell carcinoma.
    B   It spreads to the lumbar spine and the sacrum.
    C   Bone metastases are seen as osteolytic areas.
    D   Normal PSA (prostate-specific antigen) level excludes the existence of malignancy.
    E   Radical prostatectomy is the treatment of choice in all cases.

(Answers overleaf)

18.17 A False Most of the prostatic tissue lies behind the urethra. The anterior lobe in front of the urethra is very small. The prostate is also traversed by the two ejaculatory ducts.

B False Approximately 25% of the prostate is smooth muscle tissue. The smooth muscle content of a hyperplastic prostate is about 40%.

C True These vertebral veins (Batson's veins) are valveless.

D True The groove is obliterated when the prostate enlarges.

E True The posterior lobe lies inferior to the plane traversed by the ejaculatory ducts, and the lateral lobes are on either side of the median groove.

18.18 A False They are adenocarcinomas, mostly developing in the peripheral zone of the prostate.

B True Prostatic veins are connected to the vertebral venous plexus through which the tumour metastasizes. Through blood, it also spreads to liver and lungs. It also spreads through lymphatics into the pelvic and para-aortic nodes. Direct spread can involve the urethra, bladder and seminal vesicle.

C False They are osteosclerotic lesions.

D False The test has a low sensitivity and specificity. Normal levels do not rule out the existence of tumour. PSA levels can be raised by prostatic instrumentation and urinary infection. However, if the PSA levels are markedly raised, diagnosis of malignancy is more likely. Final diagnosis is done by needle biopsy and histology.

E False Radical prostatectomy should be done in patients who are likely to live for at least 10 years. If the tumour is advanced or metastatic, hormonal treatment is recommended.

18.19 Regarding carcinoma of the testis:
A   Seminomas and teratomas are more common than non-germ-cell tumours.
B   They are rarely bilateral.
C   They have an increased incidence in undescended testis.
D   α-fetoprotein and β-human chorionic gonadotrophins are tumour markers.
E   The treatment of choice is radical orchidectomy.

18.20 Regarding the scrotum and scrotal swellings:
A   The scrotum is supplied anteriorly by the ilioinguinal nerve.
B   Primary hydrocele is of congenital origin.
C   A young man with a hydrocele should have an ultrasound scan.
D   Torsion of the testis may need surgical exploration.
E   A patient over the age of 40 with a left-sided varicocele should have an ultrasound scan of the kidney.

18.21 Regarding the female genital tract:
A   Ovarian malignancy commonly spreads to the contralateral ovary.
B   The ureter lies close to the supravaginal cervix.
C   Cervical carcinoma can cause death due to uraemia.
D   Endometrial carcinoma most commonly occurs in the sixth decade.
E   Ectopic pregnancy commonly occurs in the ovary.

(Answers overleaf)

18.19 A   True   90–95% of tumours are germ cell tumours (seminomas and teratomas). Seminomas have a peak incidence in the 35–40 age group whereas teratomas affect younger men (25–35 years).

B   False   Lymphomas affect men aged over 50 years and are often bilateral.

C   True   Men who have had undescended testis have a greater chance of developing testicular tumours than those with normally descended testis.

D   True   These should be estimated prior to orchidectomy. Staging is done by serological tests and CT scanning of the abdomen for lymph node metastasis.

E   True   To prevent manipulation of the testis and dissemination of tumour cells, the spermatic cord is clamped at the superficial inguinal ring prior to orchidectomy. Orchidectomy is followed by radiotherapy and chemotherapy.

18.20 A   True   It is supplied by the ilioinguinal nerve (L1) anteriorly and branches of the pudendal nerve (S2, S3) posteriorly.

B   False   Primary or idiopathic hydrocele occurs in the older age group (over 40 years). A congenital hydrocele has a hernial sac (processus vaginalis) and is connected to the peritoneal cavity.

C   True   It can be a secondary hydrocele associated with a testicular tumour.

D   True   If the treatment is delayed, infarction of the testis can occur. Absorption of dead spermatozoa may result in development of anti-sperm antibodies causing reduction in fertility.

E   True   The varicocele could be due to renal cell carcinoma spreading to the left renal vein.

18.21 A   True   It also spreads to the peritoneal cavity and the para-aortic lymph nodes.

B   True   At this level the ureter lies below the uterine artery (water under the bridge) and can be injured during hysterectomy.

C   True   Ureteric obstruction by the tumour leads to renal failure.

D   True   It has a higher incidence in nulliparous women.

E   False   It occurs commonly in the Fallopian tube.

Index

Note: references are to chapter or question and answer numbers, rather than page numbers.